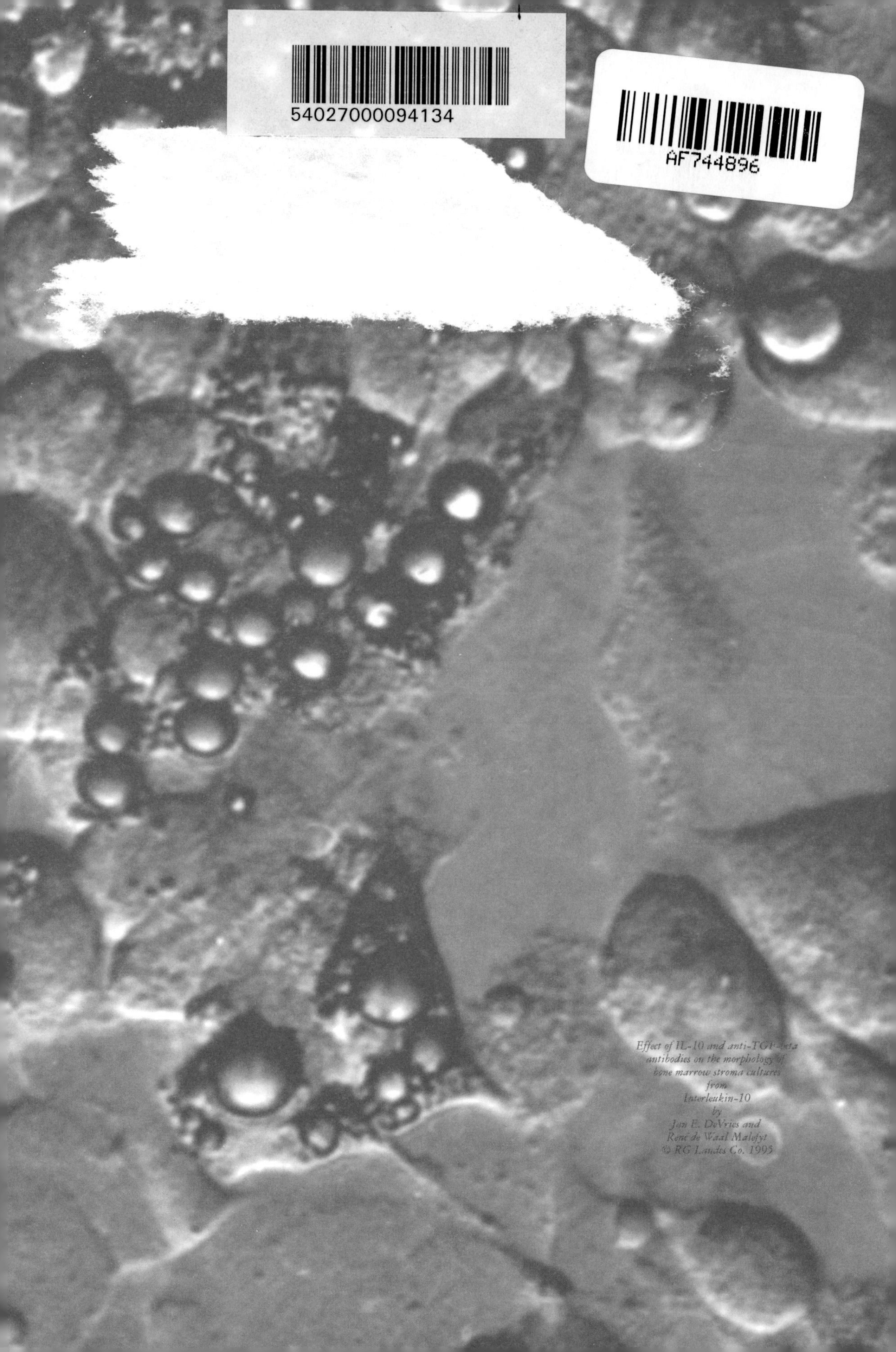

Effect of IL-10 and anti-TGF-beta antibodies on the morphology of bone marrow stroma cultures
from
Interleukin-10
by
Jan E. DeVries and René de Waal Malefyt

Molecular Biology Intelligence Unit

Antibody Therapeutics

William J. Harris, Ph.D.

Department of Molecular and Cell Biology
Marischal College
University of Aberdeen
Aberdeen, Scotland

Charles Cunningham, Ph.D.

Department of Molecular and Cell Biology
Marischal College
University of Aberdeen
Aberdeen, Scotland

Springer
New York Berlin Heidelberg London Paris
Tokyo Hong Kong Barcelona Budapest

R.G. Landes Company
Austin

Molecular Biology Intelligence Unit

ANTIBODY THERAPEUTICS

R.G. LANDES COMPANY
Austin, Texas, U.S.A.

Submitted: March 1995
Published: May 1995

Please address all inquiries to the Publisher:
R.G. Landes Company, 909 Pine Street, Georgetown, Texas, U.S.A. 78626
or
P.O. Box 4858, Austin, Texas, U.S.A. 78765
Phone: 512/ 863 7762; FAX: 512/ 863 0081

U.S. and Canada ISBN 1-57059-272-1

International ISBN 3-540-59491-4

Library of Congress Cataloging-in-Publication Data

Harris, W.J. (William J.)
Antibody therapeutics / by W.J. Harris and C. Cunningham.
p. cm. – (Molecular biology intelligence uniy)
Includes bibliographical references and index.
ISBN 1-57059-272-1 (alk. paper)
1. Immunoglobulins—Therapeutic use. 2. Monoclonal antibodies—Therapeutic use.
I. Cunningham, C. (Charles) II. Title. III. Series.
[DNLM: 1. Immunoglobulins. 2. Antibodies, Monoclonal—immunology.
3. Antibody Formation. QW 601 H317a 1995]
RM282.I44H37 1995
615'.37—dc20
DNLM/DLC 95-12615
for Library of Congress CIP

PUBLISHER'S NOTE

R.G. Landes Company publishes five book series: *Medical Intelligence Unit, Molecular Biology Intelligence Unit, Neuroscience Intelligence Unit, Tissue Engineering Intelligence Unit* and *Biotechnology Intelligence Unit.* The authors of our books are acknowledged leaders in their fields and the topics are unique. Almost without exception, no other similar books exist on these topics.

Our goal is to publish books in important and rapidly changing areas of medicine for sophisticated researchers and clinicians. To achieve this goal, we have accelerated our publishing program to conform to the fast pace in which information grows in biomedical science. Most of our books are published within 90 to 120 days of receipt of the manuscript. We would like to thank our readers for their continuing interest and welcome any comments or suggestions they may have for future books.

Deborah Muir Molsberry
Publications Director
R.G. Landes Company

CONTENTS

PREFACE

The last decade of the 19th century heralded the discovery of the existence of natural components in serum which protect and treat disease. The elements were described as 'anti-toxins' or anti-bodies ('anti-korper'). Great excitement was aroused by the possibility of using these molecules to treat disease and there has long been speculation that they could be manipulated in the laboratory as 'magic bullets'. The last decade of the 20th century is finally providing the realization of these ambitions. This book traces that journey.

Enthusiasm arising from the preliminary success of 'serum therapy' in the early 1900s was quickly muted. It was found that serum from animals had unpleasant side effects and could kill as well as cure. Life-saving cures were effected against infectious disease particularly during the first world war but patients also died from anaphylactic shock brought on by the human body recognizing animal serum as foreign.

The clinical use of human sera began in 1944 and was effective but it carried a risk of viral contamination. In 1946, a method was finally developed which effectively removed viral contamination and the immunotherapeutic product standard immune globulin (also termed immune serum globulin) was provided. This product can be given intramuscularly but it is highly viscous and causes cardiovascular and pyrogenic effects if given intravenously. Finally, in the 1970s a method for the delivery of intravenous immunoglobulin (IVIG) was developed and this product is now used in a variety of clinical situations.

It was soon realized that IVIG could be much more effective if the concentration of 'disease active' antibodies in serum preparations could be increased. Rapid and more sensitive methods for routine screening of levels of antibodies against specific disease targets have evolved in the 1980s (principally with the availability of monoclonal antibodies) and this has allowed the pre-selection of donors for inclusion in 'hyperimmune sera' which is custom designed to treat a particular disease. Chapter 3 of this book focuses on the scope and limitations of such polyclonal antisera.

Human immune sera is expensive to collect and purify and its safety is governed by the state of our knowledge of contaminants. Also, the breadth of disease against which it will be effective is limited by the protective antibodies present which in turn is decided by the diseases to which donors have been exposed. In 1975 Kohler and Milstein developed the 'hybridoma technology' which allowed the laboratory production of essentially unlimited quantities of rodent monoclonal antibodies. A monoclonal antibody against virtually any target antigen can be derived by immunization of a mouse with the antigen. By the mid 1980s thousands of rodent monoclonal antibodies against cancer cells, infectious disease targets and human tissue components, had been made and some had been shown to target and treat disease in animals. Several hundred have been used in human clinical studies and these are summarized in chapter 4.

It was assumed in 1975 that the hybridoma technology would quickly be adapted to provide a plethora of human monoclonal antibodies for a new generation of antibody based therapeutics. However this hope did not materialize and chapter 5 overviews progress which has been made towards this goal.

The era of genetic engineering has arisen from the rapid discovery of a range of novel techniques in molecular biology including rapid gene isolation, DNA sequencing, high resolution X-ray and NMR structural analysis and computer graphic 3D structure modeling of proteins and protein engineering. Chapters 1 and 2 describe their impact upon our understanding of antibody structure and function. Moreover this knowledge and these technologies came together in 1986 to allow the conversion of any rodent monoclonal antibody into an antibody of at least 95% human structure. This technique has overcome limitations on the human in vivo use of rodent monoclonals and opens the way for the exploitation of many existing rodent monoclonals as human therapeutics. The derivation and progress into the clinic of this important group of 'humanized' antibodies is described in chapter 6.

The early 1990s have also now presented us with a number of new technologies for isolating and/or design of human-like antibodies which can be derived from bacteriophage antibody display libraries (chapter 7) or transgenic mice (chapter 8). These sophisticated advances in molecular biology provide great opportunities and choice for new ways to therapeutics but they need to be assessed in the background of our current relatively rudimentary knowledge of molecular immunology.

Progress towards the goal of effective antibody based therapeutics and their use as magic bullets has been dramatic in the last ten years, with first products entering the clinic. The ultimate aim of providing custom built antibodies which seek out and destroy disease targets, and are at the same time safe, devoid of toxic side effects and immunosilent in the human body should be achievable by the end of this century. Chapter 9 overviews the new up and coming technologies and the problems which remain to be addressed.

CHAPTER 1

The Structure of Antibodies

INTRODUCTION

Immunoglobulins (antibodies) are proteins produced by B cells in response to contact with foreign antigens. They are found primarily in serum as a population of molecules separable into five major classes termed immunoglobulin A (IgA), IgE, IgG, IgD and IgM. Each class fulfills a different and characteristic function and the general properties of each class is described in Table 1.1.

Though the five classes of immunoglobulin have differing physico-chemical properties, they have the same basic subunit structure consisting of two identical light and two identical heavy polypeptide chains. Figure 1.1 is a schematic of an IgG molecule showing the light and heavy chains held together by intra- and inter-chain disulfide bonds. Each chain has a variable and a constant region with the tertiary structure of the variable region providing the binding site for antigen and the specificity of antibody binding. Each antibody molecule has, therefore, two antigen binding sites.[1]

The class of an immunoglobulin is determined by the nature of its heavy chain and the length of the hinge region (Tables 1.1 and 1.2).[2] Since these class differences are located in the constant region, the variable regions are independent of the immunoglobulin class. On the other hand, the functional properties of complement activation and Fc receptor binding reside in the constant

Table 1.1. Structural properties of human immunoglobulin classes

Property	IgG_1	IgG_2	IgG_3	IgG_4	IgM	IgA_1	IgA_2	sIgA	IgD	IgE
Heavy chain	$\gamma 1$	$\gamma 2$	$\gamma 3$	$\gamma 4$	$\mu 1$	$\alpha 1$	$\alpha 2$	$\alpha 2$	δ	ε
M.W. ($x10^3$)	146	146	170	146	970	160	160	385	184	188
Carbohydrate (%)	2-3	2-3	2-3	2-3	12	7-11	7-11	7-11	9-14	12
Half-life (days)	21	20	7	21	10	6	6	-	3	2
Intravascular distribution (%)	45	45	45	45	80	42	42	trace	75	50

Adapted from:Roitt IA, Brostoff J, Male D, eds. Essential Immunology, 3rd ed.: London: Mosby, 1993:4.1-4.19.

Table 1.2. Properties of immunoglobulin G subclasses

Property	IgG_1	IgG_2	IgG_3	IgG_4
% Total IgG in adult	60-70	20-30	5-10	<5
No. interchain disulfide bonds	2	4	11	2
No. amino acids in hinge	15	12	62	12
Biological (relative) activity -				
Complement activation	6	1	40	0
Fc receptor binding;				
Mononuclear cells	2+	1+	2+	+/-
Neutrophils	2+	+/-	2+	1+

Adapted with permission from: Hamilton RG. Human IgG subclass measurements in the clinical laboratory. Clin Chem 1987; 33:1707-1725.

regions and account for the differing biological activities of the different classes.

An IgG molecule can be dissected at the hinge region by enzymatic cleavage to yield one Fc and two Fab fragments (Fig. 1.1). Each Fab consists of an intact light chain linked to the N-terminal domain of a heavy chain and retains an antigen binding domain. The Fc fragment contains the C-terminal domains of the two heavy chains.

The major properties of each of the human immunoglobulin classes are outlined below.

Immunoglobulin G

IgG is the major immunoglobulin in serum. It represents about 80% of all immunoglobulin in normal serum and is present in

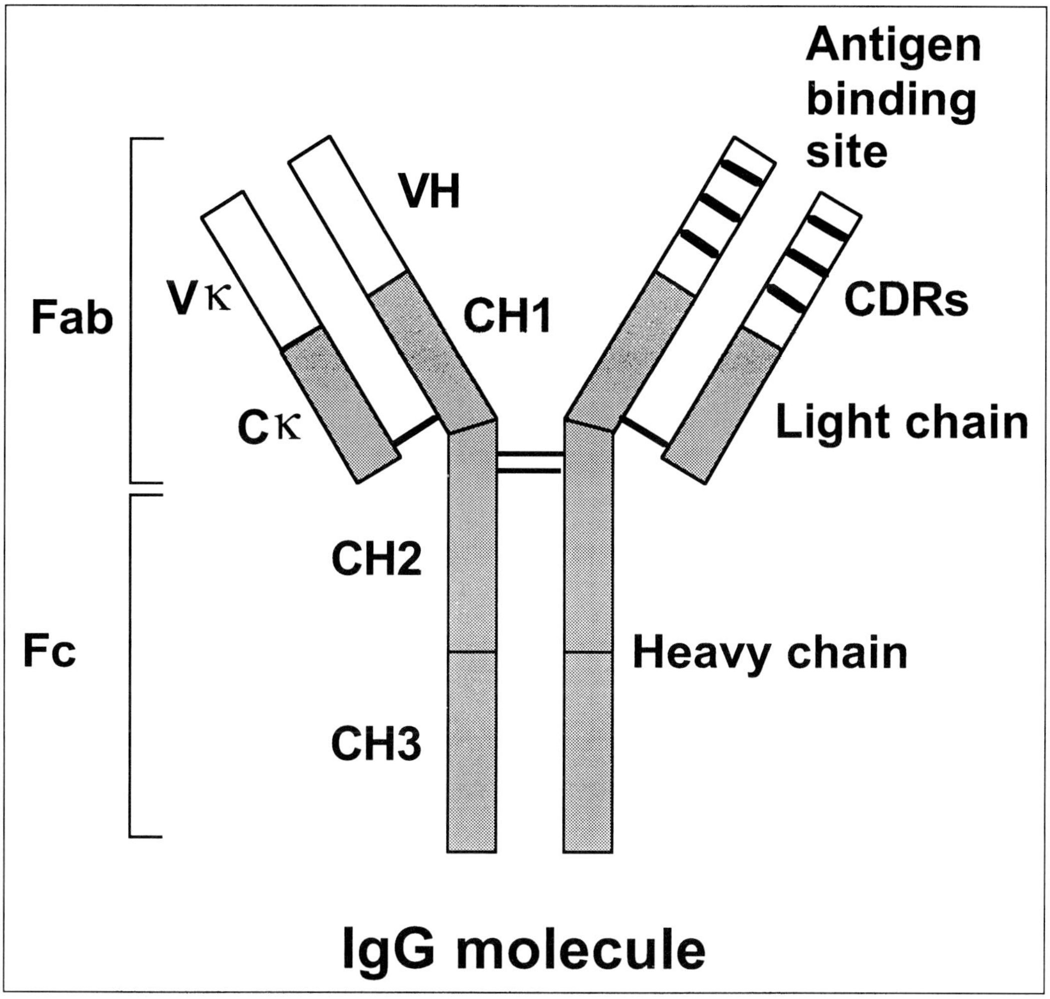

Fig. 1.1. Schematic structure of an IgG molecule consisting of two heavy chains and two light chains held together by H-bonding. Each polypeptide chain contains a variable (open boxes) and a constant (shaded boxes) region. Those heavy and light chain domains making up the Fv, Fab and Fc regions are indicated. Adapted with permission from: Zuckier LS, Rodriguez LD, Scharff D. Immunologic and pharma-cologic concepts of monoclonal antibodies. Sem Nuc Med 1989; XIX:166-186, © WB Saunders & Co., Orlando.

concentrations of 8-16 mg/ml, has a molecular mass of 150,000 daltons and has two antigen binding sites. There are four subclasses of IgG in humans (IgG_1-IgG_4) which account for 66%, 23%, 7% and 4% of the total IgG.[1] Each subclass differs in the structure of the Fc fragment, the length of hinge region, the amino acid composition of the second (CH2) and third (CH3) heavy chain constant region domains and in the degree of heavy chain domain glycosylation (Table 1.1). These differences bestow each subclass with variation in the efficiency with which they participate in activation of the antibody effector functions of complement fixation, macrophage binding and activation of cytotoxic cells through Fc receptor I (FcRI), FcRII and FcRIII. Table 1.2 summarizes the biological functions of the different immunoglobulin subtypes.

The IgG molecule is principally responsible for neutralizing infection, it diffuses into extravascular tissue more readily than the other immunoglobulin classes and crosses the placenta to provide protection to neonates. IgG molecules are, therefore, usually the antibodies of choice as therapeutics.

Immunoglobulin M

IgM is a 900,000 dalton pentamer with five IgG-like subunits held together by intramolecular disulfide bonds and is stabilized by a polypeptide anchor (termed the J-chain). It comprises 5-10% of circulating immunoglobulins and is present in serum at a concentration of 1-2 mg/ml. Due to its large size, it is confined to the intravascular space. It binds complement and as a result of its multivalency is an extremely efficient agglutinin. It is the first antibody produced in response to a foreign antigen, though usually it has a lower affinity for antigen compared with IgG. Monoclonal IgM antibodies are often produced by hybridomas and most human monoclonal antibodies are of this class. Owing to their large size, IgM molecules are more difficult to manufacture as therapeutics and their lower affinity makes them less effective than IgG molecules.

Immunoglobulin A

IgA occurs as a 160,000 dalton monomer in sera and comprises about 10-15% (1.4-4 mg/ml) of total serum immunoglobulin. Dimeric IgA is formed by the association of two monomers through a glycoprotein secretion unit. This dimeric molecule is also known as secretory IgA (sIgA) and is the predominant immunoglobulin in mucosal secretions. It binds complement and phagocytes and plays a critical role as the first line of defense against respiratory, intestinal and genitourinary tract pathogens. Methods to produce genetically engineered IgA molecules in vitro have been developed recently and therapeutics may be developed in the future.[3]

IMMUNOGLOBULIN D

IgD is a monomer of 180,000 daltons which is present in sera in varying levels from 0 to 0.4 mg/ml. It is very susceptible to proteolysis and has a half-life of only a few days. Since it does not fix complement or bind to phagocytes it is unlikely to have a protective role. It is found predominantly on the surface of B lymphocytes and probably has a role in activation and affinity maturation of B cells.

IMMUNOGLOBULIN E

IgE is a monomer of 200,000 daltons and is usually present in very low concentrations (approximately 250 ng/ml) in sera. It has a high affinity for mast cells and basophils through Fc receptor binding and stimulates an acute inflammatory response through triggering the release of cytokines and chemoeffectors.

FINE STRUCTURE OF IMMUNOGLOBULINS

Antibody structure has been intensively studied over the last thirty years and crystallographic data is now available for over 50 different antibody fragments.[4] In addition, the amino acid and nucleotide sequences have been determined for many hundreds of different antibodies from a variety of species.[5] It is only recently, however, that important advances in understanding the molecular basis of antigen-antibody interactions have been made. This understanding is crucial to the provision of novel antibody based human therapeutics.

The three dimensional structure of a typical IgG molecule consists of six discrete domains, each of which forms a compact globular structure with a characteristic fold termed the immunoglobulin fold.[6] Each domain consists of a stable arrangement of hydrogen bonded anti-parallel β sheets which form a bilayer structure stabilized by a disulfide bond between the two layers.

In the variable domains the bilayer structure is formed by nine strands. In the constant domains it is formed by seven strands. Homologous domains from different species are very similar and even when there is as much as 30% difference in amino acid sequence between two antibodies the three dimensional domain structures are essentially superimposable. Differences in structure are almost entirely confined to hypervariable regions (see below). The antigen binding region, also termed the Fv, is located on the

N terminal domain (Fig. 1.1). It has been shown in recent years that the three dimensional structure of the antigen binding domain is essentially retained intact when the antibody is fragmented into Fab or Fv fragments.[7]

It is this conservation of antibody structure, and in particular that of the antigen binding domain, which has provided the basis for the recent success of genetic and protein engineering in the development of novel antibody therapeutics.

STRUCTURE AND ASSEMBLY OF FV FRAGMENTS

Fv fragments consist of the N terminal 130 amino acid residues of each of the variable heavy (VH) and light (VL) chains held together by non-covalent interactions. VH and VL domains are synthesized in vivo by the assembly of individual gene segments, heavy chain being derived from VH, D and JH gene segments and light chain from Vκ and Jκ or Vλ and Jλ gene segments[8] (Figs. 1.2a and 1.2b). In the human genome there are 46 functional VH, at least 15 D and 6 functional JH segments, 35 functional Vκ segments, 5 functional Jκ segments and approximately 60 Vλ segments.[9] The many hundreds of immunoglobulin variable domain amino acid sequences within data bases is evidence of the diversity of the immunoglobulin repertoire. The 46 human VH gene segments are classified into seven families (Table 1.3) on the basis of nucleotide sequence homology.[10] The 32 Vκ segments are also classified into seven families.[11]

Table 1.3. Distribution of functional and pseudo germline VH and Vκ genes between human families

Family Subgroup	Number of Germline Genes			
	VH		Vκ	
	Functional	Pseudo	Functional	Pseudo
1	8	6	17	12
2	3	1	9	18
3	22	26	7	7
4	10	2	1	0
5	1	1	1	0
6	1	0	0	3
7	1	5	0	1
Total	46	41	35	41

Adapted from: Cook GP, Tomlinson IM, Walter G et al. A map of the human immunoglobulin VH locus completed by anaylsis of the telomeric region of chromosome 14q. Nature Genetics l994; 7:162-168 and Schable KF, Zachau H-G. The variable genes of the human immunoglobulin kappa locus. Biol Chem Hoppe-Seyler 1993; 374:1001-1022.

The VH and Vκ/λ gene segments provide the first 85-95 amino acids of the heavy and light chain variable domains, the remainder being from the D-J or J segments respectively (Figs. 1.2a and 1.2b). By comparing the linear amino acid sequences of many antibodies, Wu and Kabat[12] assigned the residues in Fv domains as belonging to either hypervariable regions (also termed

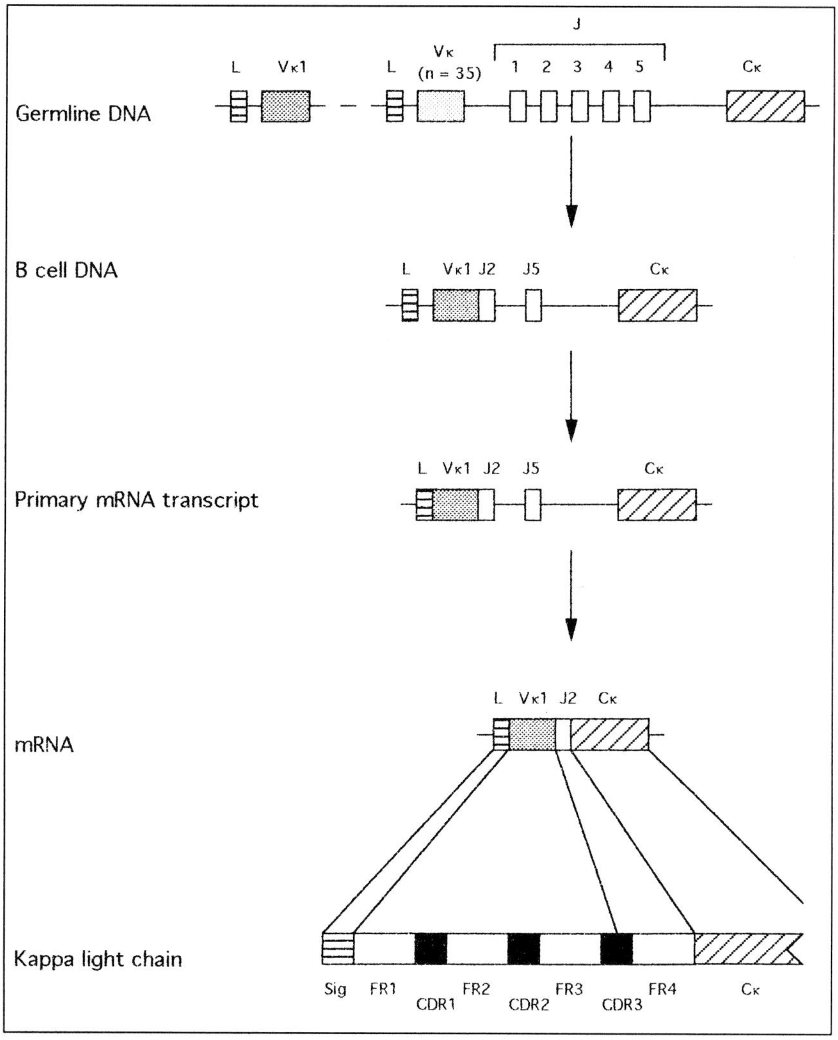

Fig. 1.2a. Assembly of Vκ gene from germ line gene segments. Germline DNA contains a tandem array of Vκ modules each consisting of a leader sequence (L) and a Vκ unit encoding the N terminal 95 amino acids. Five 'joining' (J) segments are located between the Vκ module and the Cκ segments. A Vκ and J segment are joined together by recombination to generate the reading frame for the entire light chain variable region. CDR1 and CDR2 are provided by the Vκ gene segment and CDR3 is derived from the J segment and recombination site. Adapted from: Roitt IA, Brostoff J, Male D, eds. Essential Immunology, 3rd ed.: London: Mosby, 1993:4.1-4.19.

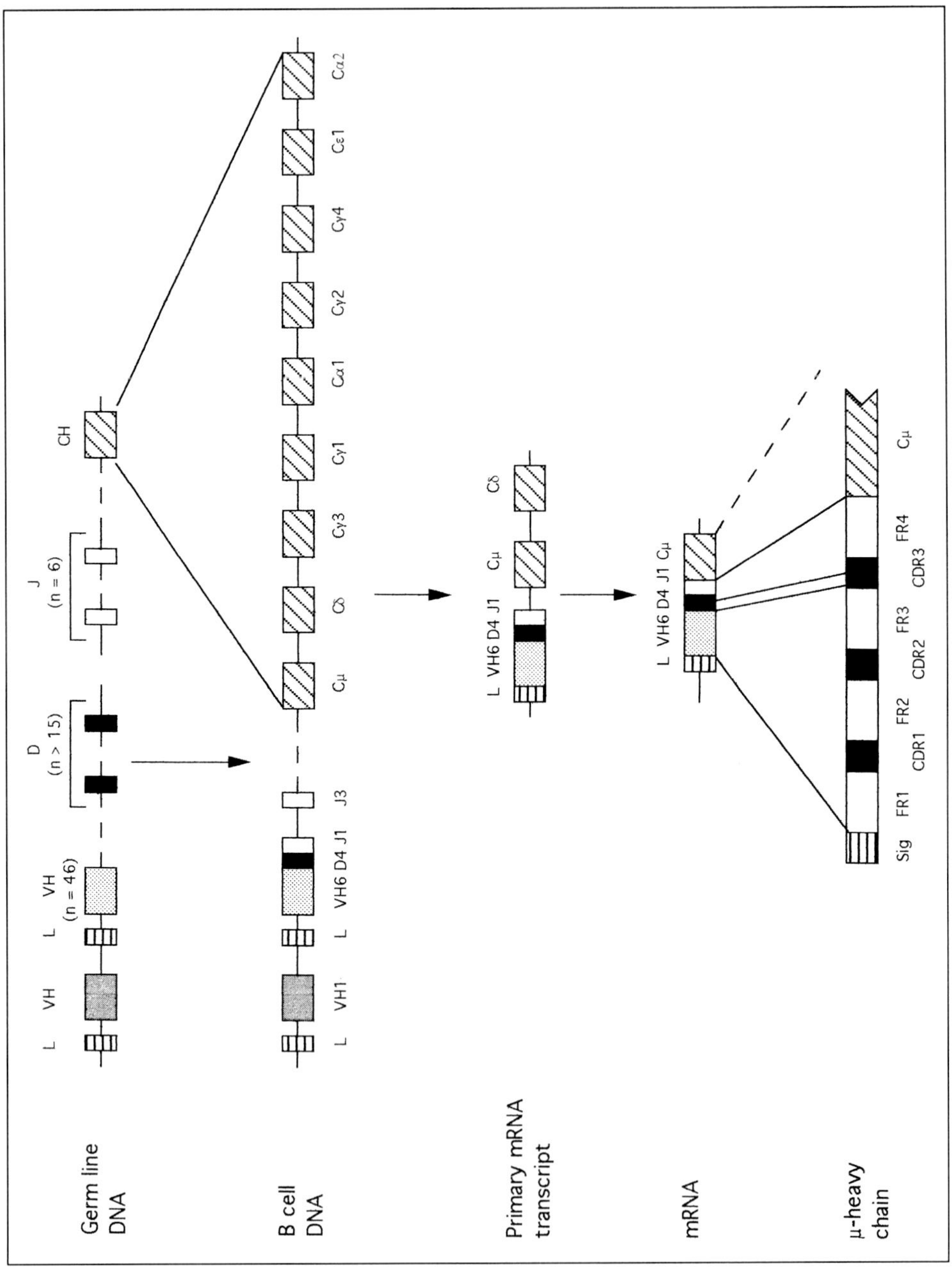

Fig. 1.2b. Assembly of VH gene from germ line gene segments. Germline DNA contains a tandem array of VH modules each consisting of a leader sequence (L) and VH module encoding the N terminal 95 amino acids. The gene for the complete heavy chain variable chain is assembled by sequential V-D and VD-J recombination events. CDR1 and CDR2 are provided by the VH gene segment and CDR3 results from the VDJ recombination site. Adapted from: Roitt IA, Brostoff J, Male D, eds. Essential Immunology, 3rd ed.: London: Mosby, 1993:4.1-4.19.

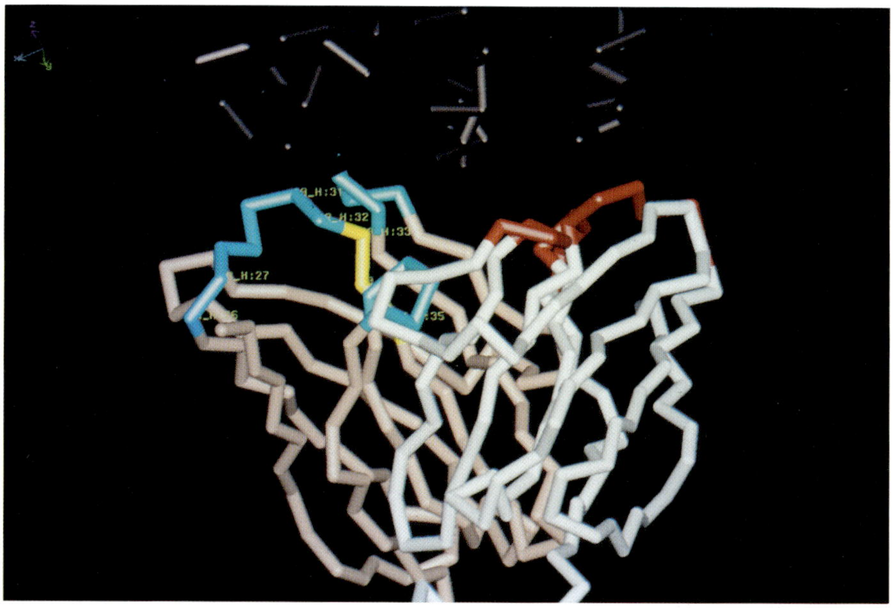

Fig. 1.3. A 3D computer graphic model of Fv segment of an anti-lysozyme antibody. VH (pink) and Vκ (white) are shown with the individual loops of the VH domain (blue) and the Vκ domain (red). The yellow segment highlights the amino acid residues which are included in CDR1 though they lie without loop H1. The antigen is illustrated at the top of the picture.

complementarity determining regions or CDRs) or non-hypervariable framework (FR) regions. The CDRs of the human light chain are defined as residues 24-34 (CDR1-L), 50-56 (CDR2-L) and 88-97 (CDR3-L). Those of the heavy chains are contained in residues 31-35 (CDR1-H), 50-65 (CDR2-H) and 95-101 (CDR3-H). CDR1 and CDR2 of both VH and VL domains are derived as a single unit from the VH or Vκ/λ germ line sequence while CDR3 is created by V-D-J (heavy chain) or V-J (light chain) joining. This joining occurs by recombination and may include genetic additions or deletions, thereby creating additional non-inherited variation in the amino acid sequence of CDR3s. Thus, CDR3-L and CDR3-H are a major source of diversity and provide individuality to different antibodies even when they are assembled using the same germ line V genes.

In crystallographic analysis, the CDRs are seen in close spatial proximity as components of loops at the N terminus of Fv (Fig. 1.3) where they create a discrete and self-contained surface.[4] In addition, these loops are fully exposed to solvent. It is this surface which is the antigen binding domain and the great variation in length, sequence and configuration of CDRs offers an infinite potential for topographical surface variation of depressions and protrusions in a 'rugged landscape'.[13] Surface variations are extensive, in some antibodies creating deep pockets, clefts and protuberances while other antigen binding sites present as gently undulating surfaces.[14,15]

VH-VL Interactions

VH-VL domain contacts vary from antibody to antibody but on average these contacts bury about 1420 Å of the surface area: 720 Å in VL and 700 Å in VH.[4] This represents about 30% of the total surface area. VH-VL domain interactions involve both framework and CDR residues with CDR participation varying from 26% to 57%. Due to the participation of CDR3 residues (Fig. 1.3), there are also significant differences in complementarity between the VH-VL domain interfaces, ranging from being better packed than protein oligomeric surfaces to being more poorly packed than antigen-antibody interactions.[16] Furthermore, VH-VL domain interfaces undergo re-alignment on binding antigen.[17] These stability factors play an important role in the selection of novel VH-VL domain combinations from immunoglobulin bacteriophage repertoire libraries (chapter 7).

Loop Structure

The six hypervariable loops (Fig. 1.3) are designated H1, H2, H3, L1, L2 and L3.[18] Of these, four are hairpins (L2, L3, H2 and H3), while L1 and H1 join one sheet of either domain to the other.

In 1992 structural data for 41 hypervariable loops from 8 different antibodies were available.[19] Analysis of this data confirmed earlier conclusions[20] and revealed discrepancies between the delineation of CDRs and the residues which make up the antigen binding loops. In CDR1-H (residues 31-35; Fig. 1.3), for example, residues 33-35 are part of the framework β pleated sheet and show little variation in three dimensional structure with residue 33 on the surface and residue 34 packed in the interior. The structural loop region is actually residues 26-32, and this is referred to as the H1 region. The main determinants of H1 structure are residue 26, a glycine, which produces a sharp turn in the peptide secondary structure and a large hydrophobic residue at position

29 that packs deep in the interior of the domain between hydrophobic residues 24 and 34. Residue 27 is also important as it packs into a surface cavity. Framework residue 94 packs against these H1 residues and affects their conformation.

Similarly, CDR2-H (residues 50-65) can be structurally divided into residues 61-65 which form part of a surface loop distant from the antigen binding site and have never been shown to interact with antigen, while residues 52-56 form an antigen binding hairpin loop referred to as H2. Framework residue 71 packs against this loop as a major structural determinant.[21]

CDR3-H varies most extensively in length and plays a distinct role in determining antibody specificity.[22] Human CDR3-H from antibodies of known specificity vary in length from 5 to 26 amino acid residues, the commonest lengths being between 10-14 residues. CDR3-H is located in the middle of the antibody combining site and its length may play an important role in fitting the contours of the antigen. With a short CDR3-H for example, the antigen surface may extend into the depression often filled by a longer CDR3-H.

CDR3-L, the C terminal end of CDR1-L and the N terminal end of CDR2-L occupy the central part of the antigen binding surface. CDR3-L, in particular, interacts with all three heavy chain CDRs with 67% of its contacts being with CDR3-H.[4] Residue 47 (usually tryptophan) in the VH domain is the only residue of the VH framework region that consistently interacts with the light chain CDRs. Specific VL framework residues which are important for CDR conformations are less clearly defined but residues within the second and fourth light chain framework regions can interact with heavy chain CDRs.

While the hypervariable loops provide the major components of the antigen binding site their conformation is altered by interaction between CDR residues and particular framework amino acids (as exampled above) and also components which determine the contacts and orientation of the VH-VL domain interface.[19-23] Framework regions do, therefore, contribute to the overall structure of the antigen binding site.

Considerable success has been achieved in recent years in the design of computer graphic models of antibodies and identification of key framework residues involved in framework-framework, framework-CDR and CDR-CDR interactions (chapter 2).

Prediction of the conformation of the CDRs proved more elusive since they occur as flexible loops which are hypervariable in amino acid sequence from one antibody to the next. However, a limited number of canonical structures have been identified for CDR1 and CDR2 with any particular canonical structure being determined by the nature of a small number of framework residues.[18] CDR3s, because of their heterogeneity, have proved refractory to accurate predictions.

The structures of antigen binding loops are therefore becoming more clearly defined, increasing the opportunity for the design of antibodies de novo (chapter 2) and a more exact humanization of antibodies (chapter 6).

Antigen-Antibody Interactions

Until recently, it was assumed that antigens bound to pockets within the antibody which had high structural complementarity to their epitope.[24] This concept was based upon early X-ray analysis of the human immunoglobulin FabNew and the study of antibodies which bound small molecular weight antigens such as phosphocholine and vitamin K1. These showed the antigen binding sites to be distinct cavities of the order of 6 Å in depth at the center of the CDRs between the heavy and light chains.[25] In recent years, however, there has been a more extensive evaluation of protein-based antigens and their interaction with antibody and this has led to the realization that the interactive surface area can be flat and undulating and occupy a considerable surface area of 2800 $Å^2$.[26] The antibody surface buried by antigen binding can vary from as little as 160 $Å^2$ for phosphocholine to 900 $Å^2$ for neuraminidase association and averages about 600-700 $Å^2$ i.e., 25% of available surface. This represents about 14 amino acids from the antibody and about the same number of atomic contacts from the antigen. Similarly, between 25% and 40% of the CDR residues contact the antigen.[4] Interacting surfaces are highly complementary in shape and charge with a packing density only slightly less than that in the interior of a folded protein.[16] Complementarity in shape has been characterized by the size of the buried surface, the packing density of interfaces and the role of water molecules. A comparative analysis of protein-protein interactions indicates that antibody-antigen interfaces have much poorer shape complementarity than oligomeric or protein-protein inhibitor complexes.[19] This is perhaps not surprising since antibodies are binding to antigens they have not previously seen in evolutionary history which is, of course, in contrast to specific protein-protein interactions which have co-evolved as an inherent part of cellular activities. This poorer shape complementarity is also likely to arise through chemical differences between interfaces. Antibodies have an above average content of aromatic amino acids in the binding site, which favors hydrogen bonding and van der Waals interactions while protein-protein interfaces are more hydrophobic.[27] Antigen-antibody interactions typically involve 9-15 hydrogen bonds and up to 3 salt bridges.[28] However, site directed mutagenesis studies infer that only a fraction of these interactions make a large contribution to binding and support the concept that there may be a 'functional epitope' in antigen-antibody interactions[29] (see loop usage below). This also supports the possibility that an antibody binding site can potentially bind several different epitopes through the use of different parts of the binding surface.

Loop Usage

In the past there has been a tacit assumption that all six loops contribute to antigen binding. However, this is not the case. The number of hypervariable loops used in binding any antigen varies from 4-6.[26] Though the number of antigens analyzed is only 14 to date, it seems that H3 and L3 are always interactive while L2 does not seem to be important for interaction with small antigens. In addition, the generally held impression that heavy chains play a greater role than light chains in antigen binding does seem to be supported by structural data.[30] Also, chain shuffling studies have shown that a heavy chain can pair promiscuously with a number of different light chains and retain antigen binding[31] (chapter 7). It is generally the central portions of loops that contact antigen; this includes the whole of CDR3-L and CDR3-H, the N terminal and middle parts of CDR1-H, CDR2-H and CDR2-L and the C terminal parts of CDR1-L.[4]

Attempts to dissect the individual contributions of antibody residues have been made through systematic calculations of the Gibbs free energy changes based on known atomic co-ordinates of antigen-antibody complexes.[29] These calculations support the view that the heavy chain and, more specifically, only a few discrete residues within each binding site contribute the significant portion of binding energies. For example, one single amino acid residue (H52) in antibody McPc 603 and three amino acids in antibody

D.1.3(H99-H101) are thought to provide the majority of binding energy. The other CDR residues contribute less binding energies and probably play an indirect role through forming the complementary shape between antigen and antibody.

These observations raise the possibility that antibody derived small peptides may retain antigen binding affinity and specificity and provide the scientific basis for much of the effort currently devoted to identifying peptide mimetics which could have therapeutic value (chapter 9).

Conformational Changes

A significant change in recent years has been the increasing acceptance that antibodies undergo conformational changes on binding to antigen. This has been demonstrated by comparison of the X-ray structures of Fabs in the antigen-bound and unbound states.[14,17,24] These analyses have included macromolecular antigens such as lysozyme and peptides and small molecular weight haptens such as progesterone, digoxin and 2-phenyl oxazolone. Such conformational changes are highly variable but can be extensive. The HIV-1 neutralizing Fab 50.1 demonstrates very large conformational changes with the H3 loop showing up to a 5.3 Å shift for main chain atoms, 6.3 Å for side chain atoms and about a 16 Å movement of the VH with respect to the VL domain.[32] Conformational changes occur in both the binding site and the overall Fv structure. The variable region is, therefore, a flexible adapter in which the VH and VL domains can move relative to each other to provide better complementarity to antigen. Thus, antibodies exist in multiple conformational states, though whether the antigen induces the change or whether there are multiple pre-existing states is still the subject of debate.[33] Though the extent to which modulation of structure can occur must be limited to preserve specificity, conformational shifts pose a new challenge to computer graphic modeling and predictive analysis (chapter 2).

CONCLUSIONS

An improved understanding of the three dimensional structure of the Fv region of antibodies has had a significant impact upon the development of antibody-based therapeutics. The appreciation of the importance of the correct conformation of hypervariable loops to antigen binding, and the importance of specific framework residues in maintaining this conformation, has been the underpinning knowledge which has allowed successful humanization of rodent monoclonal antibodies (chapter 6).

The scope and limitations of phage antibody repertoire methodologies (chapter 7) as a source of novel human antibodies depends on increasing understanding of the nature of VH-VL domain interfaces and the role of CDR3s. It remains to be seen, however, whether new opportunities for drug development will emerge from analysis of the dynamic nature of antibody-antigen interactions.

REFERENCES

1. Roitt IA, Brostoff J, Male D, eds. Essential Immunology, 3rd ed.: London: Mosby, 1993:4.1-4.19.
2. Hamilton RG. Human IgG subclass measurements in the clinical laboratory. Clin Chem 1987; 33:1707-1725.
3. Winner L, Mack J, Weltzin R et al. New model for analysis of mucosal immunity: intestinal secretion of specific monoclonal immunoglobulin A from hybridoma tumours protects against *Vibrio cholerae* infection. Infect Immunol 1991; 59:977-982.
4. Padlan EA. Anatomy of the antibody molecule. Mol Immunol 1994; 31:169-217.
5. Kabat EA, Wu TT, Perry HM et al. In: Sequences of Proteins of Immunological Interest, 5th Edition. US Department of Health and Human Services, Public Health Services, National Insitute of Health, (NIH Publication No.91-3242), 1991.
6. Poljak RJ, Amzel LM, Avey HP et al. Three-dimensional structure of the Fab' fragment of a human immunoglobulin at 2.8 Å resolution. Proc Nat Acad Sci 1973; 70:3305-3310.
7. Winter G, Milstein C. Man-made antibodies. Nature 1991; 349:293-299.
8. Honjo T, Alt FW, Rabbits TH, eds. Immunoglobulin Genes. London: Academic Press, 1990.
9. Cook GP, Tomlinson IM, Walter G et al. A map of the human immunoglobulin VH locus completed by analysis of the telomeric region of chromosome 14q. Nature Genetics 1994; 7:162-168.
10. Tomlinson IM, Walter G, Marks JD et al. The repertoire of human germ line VH sequences reveals about 50 groups of VH segments with different hypervariable loops. J Mol Biol 1992; 227:776-798.
11. Schable KF, Zachau H-G. The variable genes of the human immunoglobulin kappa locus. Biol Chem Hoppe-Seyler 1993; 374:1001-1022.
12. Wu TT, Kabat EA. An analysis of the sequences of the variable regions of Bence-Jones proteins and myeloma light chains and their

implications for antibody complementarity. J Exp Med 1970; 132:211-249.
13. Macken CA, Perelson AS. Protein evolution on rugged landscapes. Proc Nat Acad Sci 1989; 86:6191-6195.
14. Davies DR, Padlan EA, Sheriff S. Antibody-antigen complexes. Ann Rev Biochem 1990; 59: 439-473.
15. Chothia C. Antigen recognition. Curr Opin Struct Biol 1991; 1:232-236.
16. Lawrence MC, Colman PM. Shape complementarity at protein-protein interfaces. J Mol Biol 1993; 234:946-950.
17. Stanfield RL, Wilson IA. Antigen-induced conformational changes in antibodies: a problem for structural prediction and design. Trends Biotech 1994; 12:275-279.
18. Chothia C, Lesk AM. Canonical structures for the hypervariable regions of immunoglobulins. J Mol Biol 1987; 196:901-918.
19. Tramontano A, Lesk AM. Common features of the conformations of antigen binding loops in immunoglobulins and application to modeling loop conformations. Proteins: Structure, Function and Genetics. 1992; 13:231-245.
20. Chothia C, Lesk AM, Gherardi E. Structural repertoire of the human VH segments. J Mol Biol 1992; 227:799-817.
21. Tramontano A, Chothia C, Lesk AM. Framework residue 71 is a major determinant of the position and conformation of the second hypervariable region in the VH domains of immunogobulins. J Mol Biol 1990; 215:175-182.
22. Wu TT, Johnson G, Kabat EA. Length distribution of CDR3H in antibodies. Proteins: Structure, Function and Genetics 1993; 16:1-7.
23. Foote J, Winter G. Antibody framework residues affecting the conformation of hypervariable loops. J Mol Biol 1992; 224:487-499.
24. Poljak RJ. Structure of antibodies and their complexes with antigens. Mol Immunol 1991: 28:1341-1345.
25. Amzel LM, Poljak RJ, Saul F. The three dimensional structure of a combining region ligand complex of immunoglobulin NEW at 3.5 Å resolution. Proc Nat Acad Sci 1974; 71:1427-1430.
26. Wilson IA, Stanfield RL. Antibody-antigen interactions. Curr Opin Struct Biol 1993; 3:113-118.
27. Padlan EA. On the nature of antibody combining sites; unusual features that may confer on these sites an enhanced capacity for binding ligands. Proteins: Structure, Function and Genetics 1990; 7:112-124.
28. Tulip WR, Harley VR, Webster RG. N9 neuraminidase complexes with antibodies NC41 and NC10: empirical free energy calculations capture specificity trends observed with mutant binding data. Biochemistry 1994; 33:7986-7997.
29. Novotny J, Bruccoleri RE, Saul FA. On the attribution of binding energy in antigen-antibody complexes. Biochemistry 1989; 28:4735-4749.

30. Kabat EA, Wu TT. Identical V region amino acid sequences and segments of sequences in antibodies of different specificities. Relative contributions of VH and VL genes, minigenes and complementary determining regions to binding of antibody-combining sites. J Immunol 1991; 147:1709-1719.
31. Marks JD, Griffiths AD, Malmquist M. By-passing immunisation: building high affinity human antibodies by chain shuffling. Biotechnology 1992; 10:779-783.
32. Stanfield RJ, Takimoto-Kamimura M, Rini JM. Major antigen-induced domain rearrangments in an antibody. Structure 1993; 1:83-93.
33. Rini JM, Schule-Gahment U, Wilson IA. Structural evidence for induced fit as a mechanism for antibody-antigen interaction. Science 1992; 255:959-965.
34. Zuckier LS, Rodriguez LD, Scharff D. Immunologic and pharmacologic concepts of monoclonal antibodies. Sem Nuc Med 1989; XIX:166-186.

CHAPTER 2

Antibody Modeling and De Novo Antibody Design

INTRODUCTION

Recombinant DNA technology has had a decisive impact upon the pharmaceutical industry with respect to their research strategies. In particular, new drug development programs are increasingly being founded upon early identification of the macromolecular target. Putative targets normally present in cells in a few copies can be cloned and expressed in large amounts and subjected to detailed protein structure-function analysis. Mutant forms can then be generated to define biologically important epitopes. Against this background, there is increasing opportunity for the isolation and modification of antibodies or antibody fragments both as tools for the study of fine structure-activity relationships and to identify the most effective therapeutic antibody. These rational approaches are undertaken as part of design cycles[1] where both antigen and antibody can be the subject of protein engineering analysis (Fig. 2.1). Predictive modeling of the antigen binding site of antibodies can play a crucial role in such strategies.

The amount of information available through antibody sequences vastly exceeds the structural information available from X-ray analysis and neither crystallographic nor NMR analysis will become as simple and routine as nucleotide or amino acid sequencing in the foreseeable future. The major problem, therefore, is how to deduce the three dimensional structure when only sequence data is available. As databases of protein sequence have grown, it has been realized that many proteins are composed of a series of autonomously folding domains such as the immunoglobulin fold. Antibodies themselves are formed from 12 or more immunoglobulin superfamily (I) modules.[2] Thus, the most useful approach in predicting structure is through identifying common folds in proteins.[3]

Modeling of structures is essential to investigate antibody specificity for antigen, to introduce mutations to improve affinity and to design antibodies against pre-designed epitopes. The highly con-

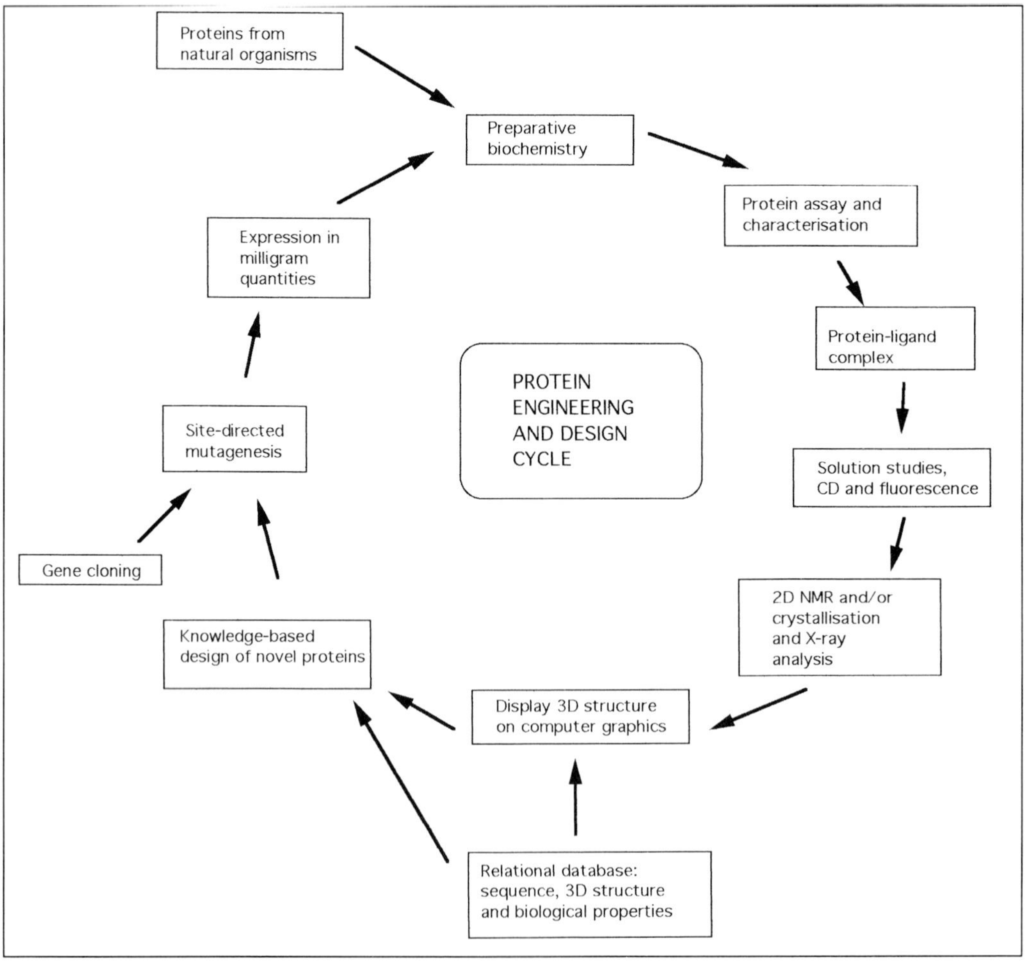

Fig. 2.1. The Protein Design Cycle. Reproduced with permission from: Blundell TL. Problems and solutions in protein engineering - towards rational step design. Tends in Biotech 1994; 12:145-148.

served structure of Fab fragments and the extensive available data bases have been used extensively to generate predictive models of antibodies. Framework regions are relatively well conserved and have proved relatively simple to model but CDRs have proved more challenging. However one can be optimistic. An important advance was the successful 'canonical' model of Chothia and colleagues[4,5] which allowed predictions of the structure of some of the antigen binding hypervariable loops. They focused on key residues at defined positions as sites which dictate CDR conformation through hydrogen bonding, packing and torsional preferences and thereby derived a limited number of alternate structures for CDR loops H1, H2, L1, L2 and L3. A very good model for the structure of these loops can be derived on the basis of size and amino acid sequence.

MODELING FRAMEWORK REGIONS

While there is promiscuity with respect to a VH domain pairing successfully with different VL domains to generate functional Fvs, the stability of such interactions varies considerably (chapter 1). This is mainly due to CDR-CDR interactions but there are also slight differences in the structure of framework regions. Analysis by Rees and colleagues[6] has shown that of the eight strands that form the central β-barrel of the Fv region there are regions of high positional conservation. Using this information, an automated VH-VL domain pairing program has been devised that allows any two variable domains to be correctly docked.[7]

MODELING CDR CONFORMATION

Two approaches have been taken to model the antibody binding site: homology based and *ab initio* (from the beginning). In the former approach the CDRs from antibodies whose crystal structure have been solved have been used to define structure on the basis of length and/or sequence.

HOMOLOGY BASED MODELING

The automated approach to homology modeling[8-10] has the following method. The sequences of the CDRs of the desired antibody are divided into a number of segments and a search is made for homologous regions from known immunoglobulin crystal structures that are most similar in size and sequence. The model is then pieced together with insertions and deletions to maximize sequence similarity. Missing atoms and inserted residues are introduced using randomized co-ordinates and the model is finalized by limited energy minimization.

While most methods use simple sequence homology to select model loop conformations, Chothia and Lesk[4] defined their canonical structures on the basis of the conservation of key residues that affect loop packing or conformation. This approach has been described in detail.[11] This is the most successful approach to date with the differences between predicted and observed structures ranging from only 0.4 Å to 3.5 Å.[5]

A major problem remains the limited data base of about 23 solved crystal structures of antibodies in the Brookhaven Protein Structural databank. An approach to overcome this limitation has been to include all protein loops described in the larger protein modeling literature.[12] This has been extended recently with the development of an object oriented data base of three dimensional structures[13] which includes information on primary, secondary and tertiary structures and additional information such as the positions of hydrogen bonds, salt bridges and disulfide bridges. This data base has been used to model the CDRs of a humanized antibody against *Clostridium perfringens* alpha toxin.[14]

Ab Initio Modeling

This approach uses *ab initio* conformational search algorithms to define all possible conformations and then selects a structure on the basis of its energy, calculated using an empirical energy function. This approach does not make use of the existing data base and is extremely consuming in computer time. Procedures for conformation generation and evaluation have been introduced into a number of computer programs.[15-17] The method of Bruccoleri and colleagues aimed to predict the structure of all six loops based on the program CONGEN.[18] All possible conformations for each loop were generated by imposing peptide dihedral angles that are energetically accessible to each residue in the sequence and sampling torsional space at 30° intervals. The number of possible structures to be screened was limited by imposing the condition that the ends of the loop should fit on to the framework with the correct geometry. The backbone differences between predicted and observed structures varied from 0.6 Å to 2.6 Å. Other methods have been reviewed.[10]

COMBINED ALGORITHMS

In this approach,[19] the above two methods are combined and exploit the structural information in the Brookhaven database and add the conformational search program CONGEN to obtain the lowest energy conformations. The conformation with the lowest hydrophobic exposed area is then selected. This has been used to model antibodies HyHEL 5, GLOOP2 and D1.3. With this approach the framework region from the Fab X-ray structure which is most homologous to the antibody of interest is used and each CDR conformation is modeled in the presence of the crystal structure of the conformation of the other five. For loops which are less than five residues in length, CONGEN alone is used while for longer loops a data base search provides candidate main chain conformations for a CONGEN-like search.

This single CDR method has now been extended and combined with the canonical structure method. For example, four or five of the CDRs are modeled with canonical structures and the remainder by the combined algorithm.

MODELING CDR3-H

CDR3-H occupies a central role in antigen binding but because of its great diversity in length and sequence it has been refractory to analysis by the canonical method. One of the factors that determines CDR conformation is the loop 'take-off' angle and through such analyses, it has been possible to define seven classes of H3 loops.[20] This has recently allowed the modeling of complete antibody combining sites with an accuracy approaching that of medium X-ray structural analysis (2.5-3.0 Å).[6] However, the recent observation that the CDR3-H loops can re-arrange on antigen binding[21,22] increases the difficulty of defining this structure.

MODELING THE ANTIGEN BINDING SURFACE

As discussed in chapter 1, the particular antigen binding moieties within the antigen binding site are made up of discrete elements which can come together to form a complementary surface and can be drawn from different parts of the surface and different parts of the loop structures. Recognition and selection of these elements offers a formidable challenge to the modeler. There does not seem to be any predictable relationship between particular combinations of CDRs or CDR lengths and antigen size except that small molecular weight haptens bind in cavities, peptides in grooves and proteins to broadly planar antibody surfaces. Predictive approaches are now being taken on the assumption that the general surface of a combining site is defined by the backbone conformation while specificity and affinity is provided by side chains.

MODELING ANTIGEN-ANTIBODY INTERACTIONS (DOCKING)

When the structure of the antigen is known, models of antigen and antibody can be constructed and attempts made to simulate their interaction. This is termed docking. Antibody-antigen interaction buries about 1500 $Å^2$ of the two surfaces. Early antigen-antibody docking simulations treated both molecules as rigid entities. Computer programs with some level of structural flexibility have recently been described but they are expensive in computational time.[21,23] A recently described method reduces the amount of configurational analysis by carrying out topological analysis of the surfaces to identify key features and then evaluates the alternate paths to linking them together.[24]

DESIGNING NEW PROPERTIES

Two properties which could have therapeutic value if built within antibodies are catalytic activity and metal binding. In the former case, the direct isolation of catalytically active monoclonal antibodies (abzymes) by traditional hybridoma methods has been under study for several years.[25] This approach is based upon the principle that immunization with transition-state analogues will give rise to monoclonals with specificity for such transition states and will *inter alia* be catalysts. Though many abzymes have been isolated their potential as therapeutics seems remote.

On the other hand, the incorporation of metal binding sites into the variable domains of antibodies has been successful.[26] Metal binding sites have been introduced into framework regions[27,28] and into CDRs using computer models which predict sites suitable for metal binding and variable region modeling[6] In one example, a tetrahedral shell of zinc was introduced through CDR1-L of an anti-lysozyme antibody. Such metalloantibodies could have potential as anti-tumor or anti-atherosclerotic agents. Semisynthetic antibody phage display libraries (chapter 7) have been constructed by Barbas and colleagues[29] by replacing CDR3-H in an anti-tetanus monoclonal antibody with a library of random amino acid sequences. From such a library they were able to isolate antibodies which bound CuII.

DESIGNING ANTIBODIES DE NOVO

It is now possible to generate relatively accurate models of antigen binding domains given the sequences of the six CDRs of an antibody. However, this is far removed from being able to predict de novo that a particular combination of CDRs will provide the correct topography for an antigen binding site. Further, the prediction of conformational changes on antigen binding has yet to be addressed in trying to predict structures with pre-determined specificity. Not only do CDR conformations need to be deduced but also CDR3-H-VH and CDR3-H-VL domain interactions.

Despite the theoretical difficulties, some progress has been made in the de novo design of an antibody combining site.[30,31] General methods have been described for assembling rigid frameworks using a common fold[32] and amino acid insertions, deletions and side chain replacements can be introduced.[33-35] Essen and Skerra[30] developed a synthetic Fv fragment which bound to chicken egg white cystatin whose crystal structure was available. In their approach, a combination of existing CDRs with a suitable backbone geometry was first selected from the data base and then different amino acid side chains were introduced to complement the precise shape and physico-chemical surface of the antigen. During the modeling, a total of 22 amino acid side chains were replaced, 12 residues in the antigen binding site and 10 residues in the framework of the Fv fragment.

Rees and colleagues[24] have suggested a strategy for remodeling a binding site to fit a different but related antigen. This is based upon the same approach of selecting an antibody from the data base with the appropriate overall topography, removing side chains from all the CDRs which are not required to define backbone structure and then replacing side chains through docking analyses.

Computer graphic analysis is greatly assisted by use of phage display techniques which allow rapid analysis of potential candidate structures (chapter 7). Of particular use are semi-synthetic antibody phage display libraries which are constructed by replacing the endogenous CDR3-H of an antibody with a library of

CDR3-Hs of random amino acid sequence and length variation. By comparing the CDR3-H amino acid sequences of phage-antibodies which bind to target antigen, one can begin to identify common key residues. Alternatively, one can include peptide motifs which mimic the natural ligand in the CDR3-H structure and randomize flanking amino acid residues with the aim of identifying phage which display the mimicking peptide in the correct conformation to bind antigen.[36]

CONCLUSIONS

Molecular models of antibody structures have been used successfully during the humanization of rodent therapeutic antibodies (chapter 6). In the future they may play an increasing role in the design of peptide mimetics of antigen binding domains of antibodies.

REFERENCES

1. Blow DM, Fersht AR, Winter G eds. Design Construction and Properties of Novel Protein Molecules. London: Royal Society, 1986.
2. Campbell ID, Downing AK. Building protein structure and function from modular units. Trends Biotech 1994; 12:168-172.
3. Taylor WR. Remotely related sequence and structure: analysis and predictive modeling. Trends Biotech 1994; 12:154-158.
4. Chothia C, Lesk AM. Canonical structures for the hypervariable region of immunoglobulins. J Mol Biol 1987; 196:901-917.
5. Chothia C, Lesk AM, Tramontano A et al. Conformation of immunoglobulin hypervariable regions. Nature 1989; 342:877-883.
6. Rees AR, Staunton D, Webster DM et al. Antibody design: beyond the natural limits. Trends Biotech 1994; 12:199-206.
7. Pederson JT, Searle S, Henry A et al. Antibody modeling: beyond homology. Immunomethods 1992; 1:126-136.
8. Anglister J, Bond MW, Frey T et al. Contribution of *trp* residues to the combining site of a monoclonal anti-dinitrophenyl spin labelled antibody. Biochemistry 1987; 26:6058-6064.
9. Levy R, Assulin O, Scherf T. Probing antibody diversity by 2-dimensional NMR: comparison of amino acid sequences, predicted structures and observed antibody-antigen interactions in complexes of two anti-peptide antibodies. Biochemistry 1989; 28:7168-7175.
10. Padlan EA, Kabat EA. Modeling of antibody combining sites. Meth Enzymol 1991; 203:3-21.
11. Lesk AM, Tramontano A. Antibody structure and structural predictions useful in guiding antibody engineering. In: Borrebaeck CAK, ed. Antibody Engineering; a practical guide. New York:WH Freeman & Co, 1981:1-38.

12. Jones TA, Thirup S. Using known substructures in protein model building and crystallography. EMBO J 1986; 5:819-822.
13. Gray PMD, Kulkarni KG, Paton NW. Object oriented databases; a semantic data model approach. Hemel Hempstead: Prentice Hall International, 1992.
14. Tempest PR, White P, Williamson ED et al. Efficient generation of a reshaped human mAb specific for the α toxin of *Clostridium perfringens*. Protein Engineering 1994; 7:1501-1507.
15. Moult J, James MNG. An algorithm for determining the conformation of polypeptide segments in proteins by systematic search. Proteins: Structure, Function and Genetics 1986; 1:146-155.
16. Fine RM, Wang H, Shenkin PS et al. Predicting antibody hypervariable loop conformations. II. Minimising and molecular dynamics studies of McPc603 from many randomly generated loop confirmations. Proteins: Structure, Function and Genetics 1986; 1:342-347.
17. Bruccoleri RE, Haber E, Novotny J. Structure of antibody loops reproduced by a conformational search algorithm. Nature 1988; 335:564-568.
18. Bruccoleri RE, Novotny J. Antibody modeling using the conformational search program CONGEN. Immunomethods 1992; 1:96-106.
19. Martin ACR, Cheetham JC, Rees AR. Modeling antibody hypervariabe loops: a combined algorithm. Proc Nat Acad Sci 1989; 86:9268-9272.
20. Searle AMJ, Pederson JT, Henry AH et al. In: Borrebaeck, CAK ed. Antibody Engineering Manual. Oxford University Press, London (in press).
21. Stanfield RL, Wilson IA. Antigen-induced conformational changes in antibodies: a problem for structural prediction and design. Trends Biotech 1994; 12:275-279.
22. Herron JN, He XM, Ballard DW et al. An autoantibody to single standed DNA: comparison of the three dimensional structure of the unliganded Fab and a deoxynucleotide-Fab complex. Proteins: Structure, Function and Genetics 1991; 11:159-175.
23. Webster DM, Henry AH, Rees AR. Antibody-antigen interactions. Curr Opin Struct Biol 1994; 4:123-129.
24. Webster DM, Pederson JT, Staunton D et al. Antibody combining sites: extending the natural limits. Appl Biochem and Biotech 1994; 47:119-134.
25. Tramontano A, Janda KD, Lerner RA. Catalytic antibodies. Science 1986; 1566-1570.
26. Iverson BL, Iverson SA., Roberts VA et al. Metalloantibodies. Science 1990; 249:659-662.
27. Roberts VA, Iverson BL, Iverson SA et al. Antibody remodeling: a general solution to the design of a metal coordination site in an antibody binding pocket. Proc Nat Acad Sci 1990; 87:6654-6658.

28. Wade WS, Jong SK, Han N et al. Engineering metal coordination sites into the antibody light chain. J Am Chem Soc 1993; 115:4449-4456.
29. Barbas CF, Rosenblum JS, Lerner RA. Direct selection of antibodies that coordinate metals from semisynthetic combinatorial libraries. Proc Nat Acad Sci 1993; 90:6385-6389.
30. Essen L-O, Skerra A. The *de novo* design of an antibody combining site: crystallographic analysis of the VL domain confirms the structural model. J Mol Biol 1994; 238:226-244.
31. Davies DR, Padlan EA, Sheriff S. Antibody-antigen complexes. Ann Rev Biochem 1990; 59:439-473.
32. Sutcliffe MJ, Haneef I, Carney D et al. Knowledge–based modeling of homologous proteins. Part 1. Three dimensional frameworks derived from the simultaneous superposition of multiple structures. Prot Eng 1989; 1:377-384.
33. Jones TH, Thirup S. Using known substructures in protein model building and crystallography. EMBO J 1986; 5:819-822.
34. Sibanda BL, Blundell TL, Thornton JM. Conformation of β-hairpins in protein structures; a systematic classification with applications to modeling by homology, electron density fitting and protein engineering. J Mol Biol 1989; 206:759-777.
35. Topham C, McLeod AS, Eisenmenger F et al. Fragment ranking in modeling protein structure: conformationally constrained environmental amino acid substitution tables. J Mol Biol 1993; 229:194-220.
36. Barbas CF, Languino LR, Smith JW. High affinity self-reactive human antibodies by design and selection: targeting the integrin ligand binding site. Proc Nat Acad Sci 1993; 90:10003-10007.
37. Blundell TL. Problems and solutions in protein engineering - towards rational step design. Trends in Biotech 1994; 12:145-148.

CHAPTER 3

IMMUNOTHERAPY

INTRODUCTION

Immunological phenomena have been observed and investigated in one form or another for many centuries. Before 1000 BC the Chinese sought protection from smallpox through 'variolation', a version of inoculation from diseased pustules and in 1796 Jenner took the rational approach of inoculating patients with material from cowpox scabs to prevent smallpox. This work demonstrated that defense mechanisms within the body were capable of being boosted and could alter the disease course.

In 1890, von Behring discovered that 'anti-toxins' were present in the serum of patients who had recovered from diphtheria and that therapy could be achieved by serum transfer. In 1900, Ehrlich defined these anti-toxins and described his 'anti-korper' theory which suggested that the body could design a range of molecules in response to foreign invasion which recognized and bound to the invading materials and effected their removal. Serum from immunized animals was then used to treat a variety of diseases in the early 1900s including pneumonia, tetanus, diphtheria and rabies. The use of human serum to treat measles, mumps and pertussis began in 1907.[1] However, serious hypersensitivity reactions were associated with the use of animal serum and the risk of viral hepatitis from convalescent human serum limited the use of serum therapy to life threatening conditions.

The gradual unraveling of our understanding that antibodies interact with foreign antigens has been accompanied by the realization that some serum antibodies can bind to other antibodies and co-exist in the same individual. These 'anti-antibodies' were first described in 1901 but it was not until 1974 that Jerne rationalized their role by formulating the hypothesis of a network of interacting antibodies through which homeostasis could be exerted to maintain a balance in the level and breadth of the specificity of serum antibodies. In particular, such immunoglobulins could exert important control over the persistence of antibodies which attack 'self' tissues. This is described as the idiotype network, with one antibody possessing a binding site (termed idiotype) which is recognized by a second antibody (termed the anti-idiotype). While each individual's serum contains a low proportion of idiotype-anti-idiotype pairs, the preponderance of such pairs is greatly increased by mixing sera from different individuals. The larger the pool of donors the greater the number of such interactions.

It is clear then that the immunoglobulin repertoire in a typical serum sample includes a wide range of antibodies with specificities against the broad range of external antigens with which the individual has come into contact. In addition, serum also contains anti-idiotypic antibodies which may recognize some of the individual's own antibodies and some from the general population.

IMMUNOGLOBULIN THERAPY

Various attempts were made in the early decades to separate the immune from the toxic serum fraction and finally Cohn and Oncley developed a procedure that recovered up to 60% of the immunoglobulin and denatured most viruses.[2] This procedure introduced standard gamma globulin (SGG), also known as immune serum globulin (ISG), into clinical use. SGG consists principally of IgG with trace amounts of IgA and IgM. Sera is pooled from approximately 1000 individuals to provide each batch of SGG and this minimizes the difference between individual antibody levels. SGG is used as a 16.5% injectable solution and represents a 20 to 25-fold enrichment of IgG found in plasma. The preparation is highly viscous and induces severe cardiovascular and pyrogenic reactions if given intravenously. It can, therefore, only be given in small doses, either intramuscularly or subcutaneously, and this limits its potential therapeutic value.

Techniques were eventually developed in the mid 1970s which concentrated intact immunoglobulin molecules and also prevented the aggregate formation which had been responsible for severe patient reactions during the pioneering use of intravenous injections.[3] This material, termed intravenous immunoglobulin (IVIG), is now used to treat a variety of diseases (Table 3.1). Commercial IVIG preparations contain about 50 mg/ml of immunoglobulin which is about five times the normal plasma concentration. A standard regime of six doses of 400 mg/kg body weight over a four week period should raise immunoglobulin serum levels by about 8 g/L with a mean half life of 20-30 days.[3] This represents about 50% of the normal serum IgG level.

Clinical use of SGG

SGG is used primarily for prevention of hepatitis A. If it is administered within a few days of exposure to either contaminated food or an infected individual it will prevent illness in 80-95% of recipients. It is also given at regular intervals to travelers to environments of poor sanitation and is used to provide some protection against non-A, non-B hepatitis and measles.[4]

Table 3.1. Successful therapeutic uses of human immunoglobulin

Standard immune globulin (SGG OR IVIG)	
Primary immune deficiencies	
X-linked hypogammaglobinemia	
Common variable immunodeficiency (CVI)	
Severe combined immunodeficieny disease (SCID)	
Secondary immune deficiencies	
Idiopathic thrombocytopenic purpura (ITP)	
Neonatal sepsis	
Malignant proliferative diseases (amelioration of secondary infections)	
Hyperimmune IVIG	
AIDS	Polio
Anti-rhesusD	Pertussis
Anti-lymphocyte immune globulin	Rabies
Anti-botulinum toxin	Rubella
Anti-*Clostridium perfringens* toxin (gas gangrene)	Tetanus
Anti-diphtheria toxin	Vaccinia
Diphtheria	Varicella
Hepatitis A and B	Human cytomegalovirus
Measles	Repiratory syncytial virus
Mumps	

Adapted from: Cross AS. Immunotherapy. In: Cryz SJ, ed. Immunotherapy and Vaccines. Weinheim: VCH, 1991:97-127.

Clinical use of Standard IVIG

The range of uses for IVIG is shown in Table 3.1.[5] A widely accepted use of IVIG is antibody replacement in immunodeficiency disease states for the prevention and treatment of infectious diseases. There is good evidence to suggest that early use in primary deficiencies can prevent much of the morbidity and early mortality in this group.[6] Despite the availability of broad spectrum antibiotics, infections are still a major cause of infant morbidity and mortality during the first month of life. Their susceptibility is likely to be due, at least in part, to a deficiency of the transfer of maternal immunoglobulin. Thus, there have been a number of studies to evaluate the use of IVIG in prophylaxis of the neonate and treatment of neonatal sepsis.[7] While the data does suggest significant clinical benefit from prophylactic treatment, evidence for therapeutic efficacy is controversial.

Secondary immune deficiencies can arise through a number of processes. Rapid excessive loss of immunoglobulin can occur in severe renal disease, gastrointestinal loss or severe burns while a shut down of B cell development with chronic lymphocytic leukemia and multiple myeloma can also cause significant depletion of serum immunoglobulin. Preliminary use of IVIG under such circumstances has on occasion shown some beneficial effect, particularly in preventing secondary microbial infections.[8] While IVIG has shown some clinical efficacy against idiopathic thrombocytopenic purpura (ITP), little or no efficacy was found during treatment of a number of other autoimmune diseases including rheumatoid arthritis, systemic vasculitis and diabetes.[8]

Anti-Infective Value of IVIG

IVIG contains a large spectrum of antibodies against a broad range of infections, which probably accounts for its general prophylactic effect in reducing infection of the immunocompromised individual. This breadth of antibody specificity is clearly of advantage under conditions where it is not possible to predict the type of infection that may be incurred. On the other hand, it is likely that the concentration of antibodies against any specific disease is severely limited and liable to be rapidly depleted by a high infective load. Under circumstances where the type of infection can be predicted it is clearly advantageous to use sera containing a high titer of antibodies against that target. For this reason, a range of high titer hyperimmune sera specific for different targets have been developed and are more efficacious than standard IVIG (see below).

Immunoregulatory Value of IVIG

IVIG exerts a range of other effects which are likely to be responsible for some of the clinical value of the preparation in secondary immune deficiencies. The large amount of immunoglobulin administered increases the level of non-specific blocking of Fc receptors on host cells. This can prevent binding of endogenous immune complexes carrying their 'pathogenic' target. In ITP, anti-platelet antibodies destroy platelets by delivering them to mononuclear phagocytes through binding of the anti-platelet antibody to the Fc receptor on phagocytes. IVIG may prevent this platelet destruction by mopping up available Fc receptors on mononuclear phagocytes.[9] Similarly, high doses of IVIG may suppress localized complement-mediated cell destruction processes through non-specific absorption of complement components.

As described above, it has been known for many years that IVIG contains dimers which arise through idiotype-anti-idiotype interactions and there is evidence that IVIG contains anti-idiotypes against some disease-specific autoantibodies.[10] These could account for the minor beneficial effects reported for some autoimmune diseases. Again, however, the concentration of any particular anti-idiotype antibody is likely to be very low.

IgM Enriched IVIG

IgM exists in serum as a pentamer with 10 antigen binding sites per complex compared with two binding sites on each IgG molecule. Because of this, complement induced lysis of bacterial cell membranes and phagocytosis can occur with approximately 1000-fold greater efficiency than through IgG. IgM enriched IVIG preparations have therefore been evaluated for general defense against infection and show some improvement over standard IVIG.[11] IgM enriched IVIG has also provided positive clinical responses when given in the early phase of septic shock.[12]

HYPERIMMUNE SERUM THERAPY

IVIG allows the administration of large volumes of antibodies directly into the blood stream to effect an immediate increase in serum levels with little pain. Recent years have also seen great improvement in diagnostic measures to screen large numbers of blood samples for high titer antibodies against specific diseases. Also, specific immunization can be used to induce an immune response in donor volunteers. A number of hyperimmune IVIG preparations are now available for specific immunotherapy against certain diseases (Table 3.1). High titer antisera is generally regarded as that which has a titer against the target which is 3-5 times above serum levels in normal healthy donors.

Hepatitis B

Hepatitis B IVIG prevents disease in 75% of people with needlestick exposure[13] and prevents transfer of the virus from mother to baby in 85-95% of cases.[14] A neutralizing human monoclonal antibody against hepatitis B is in clinical trial and has shown some efficacy (chapter 5).

Human Cytomegalovirus

Human cytomegalovirus (HCMV) is a member of the Herpes family of viruses. Infections are not usually apparent clinically but like other Herpes, HCMV persists following primary infection and may subsequently reactivate. It is widely prevalent, infecting 50-100% of adults depending on the particular population.[15] Primary infections or exacerbation of a latent infection are rare in healthy individuals but infections in patients who have undergone renal, bone marrow or cardiac transplantation are very common and are characterized by a severe clinical course. CMV infection also predisposes these patients to additional bacterial and fungal infections and increases the risk of transplant rejection. In AIDS patients, once they enter the severe immunocompromised state, CMV induced retinitis is a common occurrence.

Early clinical studies of prophylaxis in bone marrow transplant (BMT) patients with standard IVIG were disappointing though the presence of significant anti-CMV titers was not established.[16] Anti-CMV hyperimmune globulin preparations have, however, proved efficacious. Hyperimmune plasma is derived by screening donor blood and selecting those with an above normal anti-HCMV titer. Unfortunately, some commercial preparations have poor titers of neutralizing antibody and this undoubtedly accounts for some of the poorer clinical results.[17] In one study, 24 BMT patients received 200 mg/kg every two weeks after transplantation. Symptomatic infections, interstitial pneumonia and deaths were reduced.[18] Hyperimmune IVIG has been formally approved in the USA for the management of CMV infections in renal transplant patients. Human and humanized monoclonal antibodies for prophylaxis of HCMV infection are entering clinical trial (chapters 5 and 6).

Respiratory Syncytial Virus (RSV)

RSV is an important virus in the epidemiolgy of human respiratory infections causing annual winter epidemics. It is particularly serious in infants and young children causing bronchitis, bronchopneumonia and laryngotracheitis. Immunity following primary infections is usually insufficient to protect against subsequent reinfection.[19] A protective role for neutralizing anti-RSV antibodies is strongly implied by a number of studies which have demonstrated that resistance to infection or reduced severity of symptoms in infants correlated with levels of neutralizing antibody acquired by maternal transfer.[20] The anti-RSV titer in standard IVIG preparations is erratic. A hyperimmune anti-RSV IVIG (RSVIG) has been developed through pre-screening of donors for high neutralizing titer.[21] In a recently completed three year clinical trial, high risk infants and children were given once monthly doses of 500-750 mg/kg RSVIG throughout the RSV infection season and a reduction in rates of RSV infection and hospitalization was noted.[22] An application for an Investigational New Drug (IND) license for this product was recently rejected by the US FDA which is seeking further data. A humanized monoclonal antibody for prophylaxis and treatment of acute repiratory RSV infections in children is currently in clinical trial (see chapter 6).

Human Immunodeficiency Virus (HIV)

A large multicenter trial of standard IVIG in symptomatic HIV-infected children showed reduced incidences of bacterial infections and fewer hospital admissions.[23] Hyperimmune sera have been derived by pooling blood from up to 1000 donors who are HIV-positive, are at an early stage of infection and are clinically healthy. This has been used in a phase I/II study with 220 patients. Of 21 patients who received a high dose of antisera only one died during the treatment period (5%) compared with 6/30 deaths (20%) in the control group. In contrast to the control group, the treated patients also showed a recovery of levels of $CD4^+$ cells in blood.[24] Though these results fall short of statistical significance, further trials are ongoing.

Varicella zoster (VZV)

Immunocompromised children under 15 years of age, babies whose mothers develop chickenpox, premature babies whose mothers are seronegative and all premature babies of less than 28 weeks of gestation receive varicella zoster IVIG (Zig) as soon as possible after exposure to the virus. Under these circumstances it ameliorates but does not prevent infection. Due to the paucity of high titer neutralizing antisera in the population, Zig is in very limited supply and expensive. Its use to date has therefore been restricted to severe life threatening situations.[25] A potent neutralizing humanized monoclonal antibody is in pre-clinical development and this should allow much greater application in the broader at-risk populations (chapter 6).

Rabies

Anti-rabies IVIG is prepared from hyperimmunized volunteers and is used in conjunction with the human rabies vaccine to decrease transmission and death after exposure to rabid animals.[6] It is efficacious in preventing infection.

CONCLUSIONS

There is a now a considerable body of evidence that IVIG can ameliorate disease symptoms in a number of clinical situations, particularly with respect to reducing susceptibility to microbial infections. Hyperimmune sera containing a higher concentration of target specific antibodies is superior to standard IVIG in treating specific diseases. This supports the concept that antibody therapy is effective, a limiting factor being the concentration of biologically active antibody present in the therapeutic preparation. Even with hyperimmune sera, this is likely to be well below 1%. There are grounds for optimism then that monoclonal antibody based products in which 100% of immunoglobulin is directed at the disease target will be very effective therapeutics. IVIG studies have also shown that one can deliver very large doses of immunoglobulin, equivalent to 50% of normal circulating serum level, with safety and without toxic side effects. The new generation of monoclonal antibody based products can therefore be given to increase the serum content of a therapeutic antibody to unprecedented levels of up to 10,000 fold higher than the typical level in the body.

REFERENCES

1. Grabar P. The historical background of immunology. In: Stites DP, Stobo JD, Wells JV, eds. Basic and Clinical Immunology, 6th ed. Norwalk: Appleton and Lange, 1989:3-14.
2. Finlayson JA. In: Easmon CSDF, Jeljaszewicz J, eds. Medical Microbiology, Volume I. 1982:129-192.
3. Ochs HD, Buckley RH, Pirofsky B et al. Safety and patient acceptability of intravenous immunoglobulin in 10% maltose. Lancet 1980; ii:1158-1159.
4. Bean B. Antiviral therapy: current concepts and practices. Clinical Microbiol Rev 1992; 5:146-182
5. Cross AS. Immunotherapy. In: Cryz SJ, ed. Immunotherapy and Vaccines. Weinheim: VCH, 1991:97-127.
6. Cunningham-Rundles C, Siegal FP, Smithwick EM et al. Efficacy of intravenous immunoglobulin in primary immunodeficiency disease. Ann Intern Med 1984; 101:435-439.
7. Ugazio AG, Chirico G, Duse M et al. Immunoglobulin treatment and prophylaxis in the neonate. In: Imbach P, ed. Immunotherapy with Intravenous Immunoglobulins. London: Academic Press, 1991:75-92.
8. Imbach P ed. Immunotherapy with Intravenous Immunoglobulins. London: Academic Press, 1991.
9. Imbach P, Barandun S, D'ApuzzoV et al. High-dose intravenous gammaglobulin for idiopathic thrombocytopenic purpura in childhood. Lancet 1981; i:1228-1231.
10. Kaveri SV, Dietrich G, Hurez V et al. Intravenous immunoglobulins (IVIG) in the treatment of autoimmune diseases. Clin Exp Immunol 1991; 86:192-198. Erratum in Clin Exp Immunol 1992; 88:373.
11. Garbett ND, Munro CS, Cole PJ. Opsonic activity of a new intravenous immunoglobulin preparation: Pentaglobin compared with Sandoglobin. Clin Exp Immunol 1989; 76:8-12.
12. Schedel I, Dreikhausen U, Nentwig B et al. Treatment of gram-negative septic shock with an immunoglobulin preparation: a prospective randomised clinical trial. Critical Care Medicine 1991; 19:1104-1113.
13. Seef LB, Wright EC, Zimmerman HJ et al. Type B hepatitis after needlestick exposure: prevention with hepatitis B immune globulin. Ann Intern Med 1978; 88:285-293.
14. Centers for Disease Control. Protection against viral hepatitis. Morbid Mortal Weekly Rep 1990; 39:1-15.

15. Grundy JE. The biology of cytomegalovirus infection. In: Touraine JL, ed. Transplantation and Clinical Immunology XXIII: viruses and transplantation. Amsterdam; Elsevier, 1991:89-96.
16. Elfenbein G, Krischer J, Rand K et al. Preliminary results of a multicenter trial to prevent death from cytomegalovirus pneumonia with intravenous immunoglobulin after allogeneic bone marrow transplantation. Transplant Proc 1987; XIX:138-143.
17. Roy DM, Grundy JE. Evaluation of neutralising antibody titers against human cytomegalovirus in intravenous gammaglobulin preparations. Transplantation 1992; 54:1109-1112.
18. Winston DJ, Pollard RB, Winston G et al. Cytomegalovirus immune plasma in bone marrow transplant recipients. Annals Int Med 1982; 97:11-18.
19. Kim HW, Arrobio JO, Brandt CD et al. Epidemiology of respiratory syncytial virus infection in Washington DC. I. Importance of the virus in different respiratory tract syndromes and temporal distribution of infection. Am J Epidemiol 1973; 98:216-225.
20. Ward KA, Lambden PR, Ogilvie MM et al. Antibodies to respiratory syncytial virus polypeptides and their significance in human infection. J Gen Virol 1983; 64:1867-1876.
21. Siber GR, Leszczynski J, Pena-Cruz V et al. Protective activity of a human respiratory syncytial virus immune globulin prepared from donors screened by microneutralisation assay. J Infect Dis 1994; 169:1368-1373.
22. Groothius JR, Simoes EAF, Levin JJ et al. Prophylactic administration of respiratory syncytial virus immune globulin to high-risk infants and young children. N Eng J Med 1993; 329:1524-1530.
23. National Institute of Child Health and Human Development Intravenous Immunoglobulin Study Group. Intravenous immune globulin for the prevention of bacterial infections in children with symptomatic human immunodeficency virus infection. N Eng J Med 1991; 325:73-80.
24. Levy JL. Anti-HIV Hyperimmune plasma: a new weapon in the anti-AIDS armory is under trial. In: Price E, ed. The Biotechnology Report 1994/95. Hong Kong: Campden Publishing Ltd, 1994:98-99.
25. Centers for Disease Control. Varicella zoster immune globulin for the prevention of chickenpox: recommendations of the immunization practices advisory committee. Ann Intern Med 1984; 100:859-865.
26. Centers for Disease Control. Rabies prevention - United States 1984. Morbid Mortal Weekly Rep 1984; 33:393-408.

CHAPTER 4

Clinical Studies with Murine and Chimeric Monoclonal Antibodies

INTRODUCTION

A search of industrial data bases suggests that about 140 murine monoclonal antibodies were under investigation as candidate clinical products up to 1993 and about 50 had been tested in humans. Thus, at present, murine monoclonal antibodies are the major source of clinical data. The vast majority of these trials have been in less than ten, principally cancer, patients. In the future it is likely that trials with humanized antibodies will dominate but the long lead time from research to clinic ensures that the current clinical data with murine monoclonals will remain a good basis for defining the potential of antibody therapy.

A number of general conclusions are clear. No major toxicity has been observed through the use of unconjugated murine monoclonal antibodies. Major toxicity can arise, however, through conjugation to drugs, toxins or radioisotopes. The major problems in the use of rodent monoclonals are (a) a short half life which necessitates frequent and multiple dosing regimes, (b) poor recognition of murine antibody constant domains by human effector mechanisms and (c) the human anti-murine response (HAMA) which arises through the human immune system recognizing the murine protein as foreign. HAMA responses develop in about 50%

---

of patients after a single dosing and in about 90% of patients after repeat treatment, resulting in rapid clearance of antibody.[1]

In practice, therefore, any therapeutic effects reported for murine antibodies are due to the first or second doses as these are the only ones which reach the target.[2] Bearing this in mind then, the data reported below can be considered to strongly support the 'proof of principle' that monoclonal antibody therapy can be effective.

CHIMERIC ANTIBODIES

The first approach to improve upon the therapeutic efficacy of rodent monoclonal antibodies was the generation of rodent-human chimeric antibodies by genetic engineering.[3] This methodology replaced the VH and VL constant domains of parental rodent antibodies with human constant regions (Fig. 4.1). The genes for all human immunoglobulin subtypes have been cloned and it is therefore possible to construct an antibody of any required subtype. As described below, chimeric antibodies in clinical trial have improved serum half lives and reduced HAMA responses in comparison to murine monoclonal antibodies. Shortly after chimerization technology was developed it was superseded by humanization (reshaping) technology (chapter 6). However, only a few clinical trials with humanized antibodies have begun thus far though it is the preferred technology for improving the therapeutic properties of rodent antibodies.

Chimeric antibodies have, however, made several important contributions to advances in the field. A number of IgM antibodies have been developed with useful in vivo imaging properties, but imaging with the intact molecule gives rise to high background. In addition, IgM antibodies are more difficult to purify due to their tendency to aggregate. Fab or $F(ab')_2$ fragments are therefore the diagnostics of choice but such fragments are difficult to prepare by proteolytic digestion of IgM molecules. In a number of cases mouse-human IgG chimerics have been prepared to provide a molecule easily digested with trypsin or pepsin to provide Fab fragments for imaging. Such fragments also give rise to a diminished HAMA response.

Clinical trials with chimerics have shown them to be safe nontoxic therapeutics. Immune responses are reduced from being present in up to 80% of patients to as few as 5% (Table 4.1) but the residual HAMA response is still sufficient to block the clinical

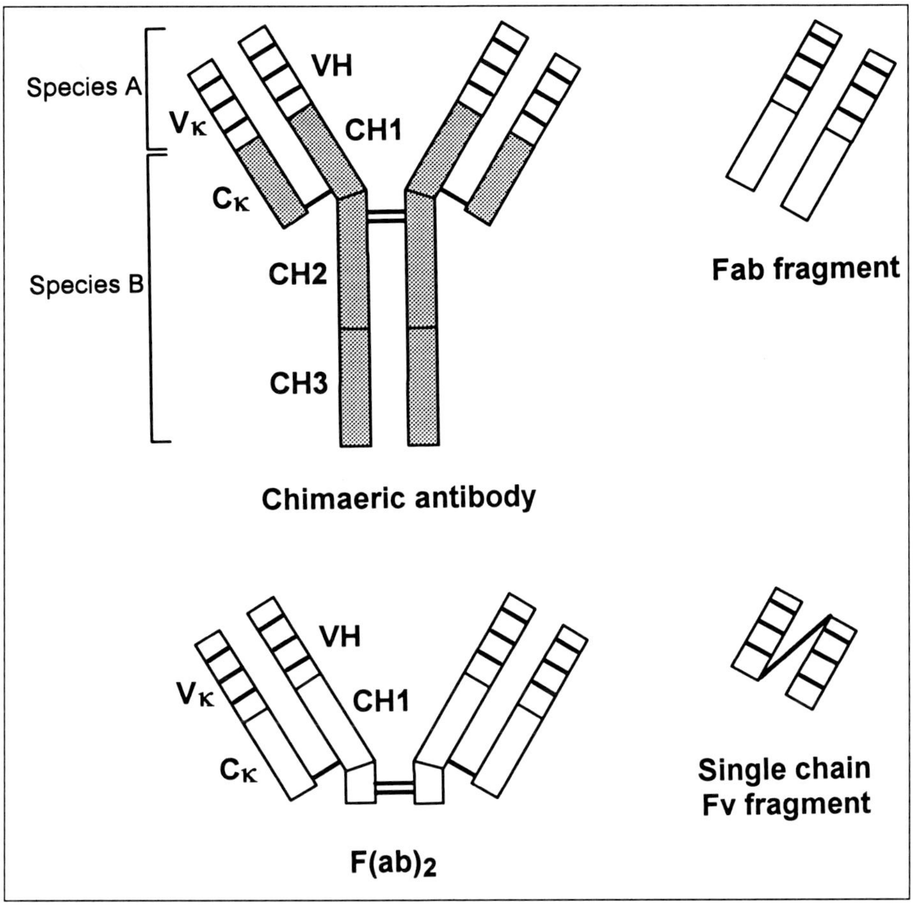

Fig. 4.1. Structure of chimeric IgG and fragments. Chimeric mouse-human antibodies are constructed by fusing the genes for murine variable regions (species A) to genes encoding human constant regions (species B). The resulting chimeric retains the antigen binding affinity and specificity of the original murine antibody but has intact human effector function activities.

Table 4.1. Comparative pharmacokinetics and HAMA response from murine and chimeric monoclonals

	Mean t1/2β (hours)			HAMA (% Patients)		
	Monoclonal antibody					
	17-1A	B72.3	L-6	17-1A	B72.3	L-6
Murine	19	42	96	80-90	70	67
Chimeric	86	230	96	5	70	25

See text for reference

efficacy of repeated dosing.[4] Analysis of the residual HAMA response has shown it to be concentrated upon the rodent Fv components. The greatly varying reduction in HAMA observed between antibodies 17-1A and B72.3[5,6] also implies great variability in the inherent immunogenicity of rodent Fv regions and opens up the possibility of pre-selecting rodent monoclonal antibodies of low immunogenicity. This data provides considerable optimism that the further reduction in rodent components in humanized antibodies will overcome the problems of HAMA responses.

PHARMACOKINETICS OF MURINE AND CHIMERIC MONOCLONAL ANTIBODIES

Typical pharmacokinetics for rodent and chimeric monoclonals are shown in Figure 4.2.[4,7] Intact murine antibodies exhibit one component kinetics with the murine t1/2 of 40-50 hours. Mouse-human chimeric antibodies have two component kinetics with a t1/2α of approximately 20 hours reflecting the initial equilibrium

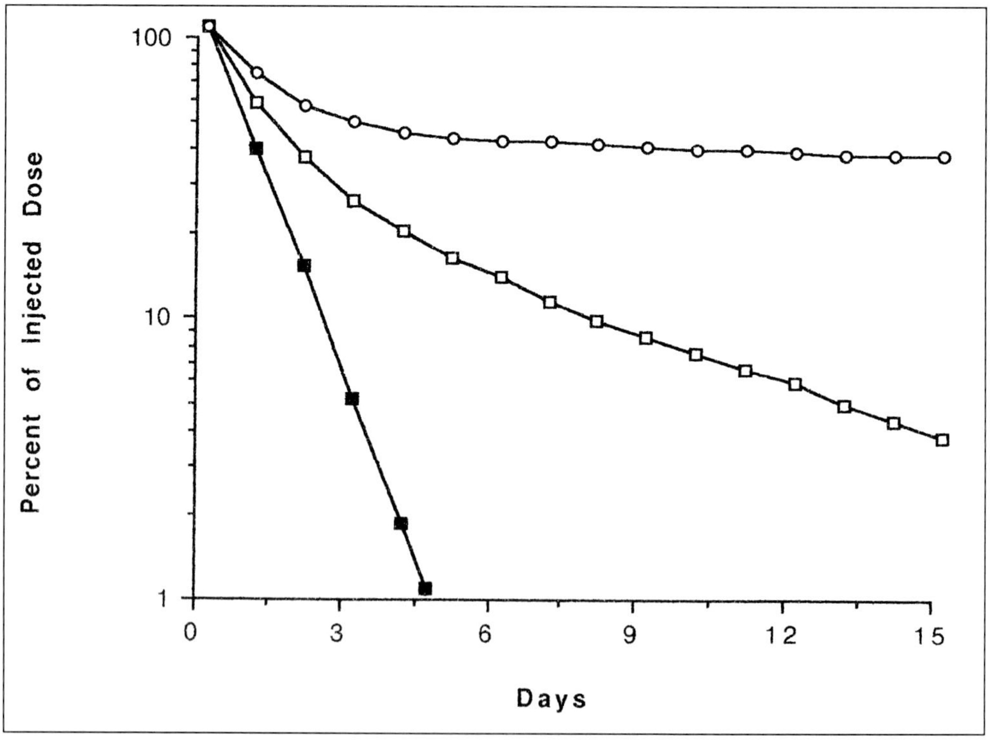

Fig. 4.2. Pharmacokinetics in man of murine and chimeric mouse-human antibodies. Typical in vivo human serum clearance kinetics of murine (■) chimeric (□) and human (O) antibodies are depicted. Adapted from: Lo Buglio AF, Wheeler RH, Trang J et al. Mouse/human chimeric monoclonal antibody in man: kinetics and immune reponse. Proc Nat Acad Sci 1989; 86:4220-4224.

between serum and tissues and t1/2β up to 230 hours reflecting serum clearance. Chimerization improves serum half-life by about 5-fold (Table 4.1) to t1/2β of 3-10 days but this is still shorter than the 14-21 days typical of human monoclonal antibodies.

Antibody fragment formulations of Fab, $F(ab')_2$, scFv (Fig. 4.1) all demonstrate a more rapid access into extravascular space and clearance from serum. These properties and their differing biodistributions and penetration into tissue or tumors is leading to their preferred use in imaging and some therapeutic applications.[8]

CLINICAL STUDIES

INFECTIOUS DISEASE

Septic shock

Murine IgM monoclonal antibody E5 (Xoma) is a murine IgM of low affinity derived from a mouse immunized with the J5 rough mutant of *E. coli*. It has undergone considerable clinical development to target the treatment of septic shock. The antibody binds to the endotoxin lipid A component of LPS of rough gram negative bacteria[9,10] and early clinical studies were interpreted to suggest that the antibody reduced mortality and enhanced the resolution of organ failure among patients with gram negative sepsis who were treated prior to entrance into a septic shock state.[11] Four hundred and eighty-six patients were enrolled in this study and received two doses of 2 mg/kg/24 hours of E5 or placebo in addition to ongoing antimicrobial therapy. Fifty-four percent of the patients were bacteremic and 46% non-bacteremic. Overall survival was not improved but the data indicated that those not in shock at entry had a 2.3-fold improved survival rate. Further trials resulted in about 1300 patients being treated and all data was pooled in to a single 'meta-analysis'. A HAMA response was found in about 50% of patients. The antibody was rapidly cleared with a half life of the order of 20 hours. Trials did not provide clear evidence of efficacy and in 1992 FDA approval was not given. Sepsis is a complex condition involving a network of interactions, and demonstrating efficacy with a single agent in broadly based trials may not be possible. E5 is currently in a more focused 1700 patient phase III trial by Pfizer in patients suffering from gram negative sepsis and organ dysfunction.

HIV

Fourteen monoclonal antibodies with promising in vitro neutralizing activity against HIV have been compared in the WHO/NIAID sponsored Antibody Serological Project (ASP) whereby samples of all monoclonal antibodies were sent to a variety of laboratories for confirmatory in vitro neutralization studies and ranking with respect to potency.[12] It is likely that the most promising of these will be selected for clinical trial in the near future. AIDS-439 (Tanox Biosystems) is an IgG1 chimeric antibody, with specificity for the V3 region of gp120, which neutralizes both IIIB and MN strains. A phase I/IIa study involved an open labeled, uncontrolled study in 12 advanced AIDS patients who received up to 20 mg of antibody every three weeks for up to six months. The product was safe with minimal immunogenicity and a terminal half-life of 1-2 weeks. There was high variability in patient responses, as measured by anti-HIV assays of p24 levels or PCR detection of viral RNA, but 3/8 patients showed a clear decrease in both assays.[13] A long term response rate of even 20-30% is promising for a single monoclonal antibody but serves to emphasize the likely need for a cocktail of antibodies for greater efficacy

CANCER

Over 100 murine monoclonal antibodies against tumor associated antigens have been described[2,4] recognizing oncofetal or tissue-specific antigens, growth factor receptors or oncogene products. Oncofetal antigens are expressed on a spectrum of carcinoma types and therefore have potential for use against tumors from a variety of organs and tissues. The initial use of such antibodies has been in the detection of antigens in serum or urine to diagnose disease and select patients whose tumors may be reactive to a particular monoclonal antibody. The most commonly used are monoclonal antibodies against the carcinoembryonic antigen (CEA) and the less well defined surface markers CA19-1, CA-125, CA15-3 and TAG-72.

IN VIVO IMAGING

Nearly 200 clinical trials of radiolabeled monoclonal antibodies for in vivo tumor imaging and targeting studies have been carried out since 1978 and such studies have helped define the opportunities and limitations of rodent antibodies for therapy. About 20 companies are committed to these studies. The leaders include

Centocor, Cytogen and Immunomedics. A list of those antibodies used in radiolabeled imaging studies is presented in Table 4.2. OncoTrac small cell lung cancer (SCLC) Imaging kit is claimed to be the most sensitive single test to determine the degree of spread of disease in small cell lung cancer patients and is at the final stage for FDA approval.

Iodine-131, Iodine-123, Indium-111 and Technetium-99 are the main radionuclides which have been used. Of these Tc99m is the preferred radionuclide because of its high-intensity photon energy, good uptake kinetics and ease of on-site generation at low cost. Tc99m conjugation chemistry is, however, less well developed and most clinical studies to date have used ^{131}I though the β-radiation of this radionuclide is more suitable for therapy than imaging. Several thousand patients have been studied by radioimmunoim-aging with 60-90% of lesions being correctly identified. Such imaging can help distinguish between a malignant lesion and a previous scar from radiation therapy or surgery and is proving particularly useful when used in combination with tomographic methods of single photon emission tomography

Table 4.2. Monoclonal antibodies used in in vivo radiolabeled imaging studies

Antibody	Antigen	Tumor	Reference
^{131}I-MN14-4	CEA	colon/lung/breast	15,16,19
^{111}In-anti-CEA	CEA	lung	17
^{111}In-B72.3:			
OncoScint CYT103	TAG-72	colon	18-20
OncoScint CYT103	TAG-72	ovary	21,22
^{111}In-7E11C5.3:			
OncoScint PR356	-	prostate/bone metastasis	23
^{99}Tc-CC49	TAG-72	colon/breast/ovary	24
^{131}I-17-1A	37 kD gp	colon	25
BCD-F9	-	breast	26
OC125	-	ovary	27
^{64}Cu-1A3	-	colon/pelvis	23
^{131}I-H17E2	PLAP	ovary	28
HMFG	mucin	ovary	29
^{131}I-p97	-	melanoma	30
^{131}I-lym-1	HLA-DR	lymphoma	31
^{99}TcNR-ML-05	-	melanoma	32
^{131}I-G250	-	kidney	33
^{99}Tc-LL-2	-	non-Hodgkin's lymphoma	24
^{99}Tc-IMMU-CEA	CEA	colon	24

(SPECT) or positron emission tomography (PET) to increase the target-to-background contrast. Tumors as small as 0.5 cm^2, which may be missed by other techniques, can be detected. More details from trials with the lead monoclonal antibodies against antigens CEA and TAG-72 are detailed below

One non-tumor target product licensed in Europe for several years is MYOSCINT for cardiac imaging and locating necrosis in acute ischemic heart disease. This anti-myosin, used as a ^{111}In labeled Fab fragment, has been employed in trials of over 1000 patients world-wide with a claimed overall sensitivity of 82% and specificity of 100%. Positive images are obtained and confirm myocardial infarction even in the absence of detectable electrocardiac changes.[34]

THERAPEUTIC STUDIES

UNCONJUGATED MONOCLONAL ANTIBODIES

The first clinical studies in the early 1980s with antibodies against lymphomas and leukemias showed transient, rapid clearance of tumor cells using monoclonal antibodies AB 89 and J-5.[35,36] Subsequent phase I and II trials have been carried out or are ongoing with at least 15 other unconjugated monoclonal antibodies (Table 4.3). These studies have shown partial clinical responses but virtually all patients developed HAMA, thus preventing repeat treatment. The studies have, however, clearly demonstrated the potential for tumor monoclonal antibody based therapy with minimal toxicity.

An anti-idiotypic monoclonal antibody was used to treat a patient with follicular lymphoma and complete remission was reported.[55] Later trials of anti-B cell lymphoma anti-idiotypes showed partial responses but tumors returned later and no longer bound to the anti-idiotype.[56] With this kind of therapy, each anti-idiotype has to be raised against the patient's own tumor cells, though some epitopes shared by B cell lymphomas from different patients have now been identified and a panel of anti-idiotypic monoclonal antibodies is being assembled.[57]

Trials have recently been initiated with bifunctional antibodies. A phase I study with antibody 2B1 (c-erbB2:FcγRIII) at 1-5 mg/ml in patients with refractory c-erbB-2 positive tumors gave preliminary indications of clinical activity but thrombocytopenia

Table 4.3. Unconjugated murine monoclonals which have been used in human cancer clinical trials

Antibody	Antigen	Tumor	Responders	Reference
AB89	-	BCL	0/1	35
J-5	CD10	ALL	0/4	36
17-1A	37 kD gp	colorectal	3/137	37
R24	ganglioside	malignant melanoma	4/21	38
NP-2	CEA	gastrointestinal	-	39
B72.3	TAG-72	peritoneal carcinoma	-	40
3F8	ganglioside gd2	melanoma	2/9	41
96.5	-	melanoma	-	42
T101	CD5	CLL	0/10	43
L17F12	-	TCL	-	44
MDX-11	-	AML	-	45
ANTI-TAC	CD25	T-ALL	6/19	46
CAMPATH-1	CAMPATH	ALL	3/5	47
L-6	CD22	non Hodgkin's lymphoma	1/14	48
Bifunctional antibodies				
2B1:				
c-erbB2 x FCγRIII	-	ovary/colon/breast	-	49
MOV18xCD3	-	ovary	-	50
MDX-210:				
(HER-2/neu x FcγRI)	-	breast/ovary	-	51
Chimeric antibodies				
B72.3	-	colorectal	-	4,52
17-1A	-	colorectal	-	4,53
C2B8	CD20	B cell lymphoma	6/15	54

toxicity was dose limiting and HAMA responses were induced in 14/15 patients.[49] Four patients had noticeable reductions in tumor load. A phase I/II clinical trial with MDX-210 (anti-HER-2/neu: anti-FcγRI (CD64)) in breast and ovarian cancer has been completed.[51] Doses of 0.35-10 mg/m^2 were used in 15 patients. Serum half life was 8-16 hours and targeting to monocytes was indicated by stimulation of the release of cytokines TNFα, IL-6 and granulocytic colony stimulating factor (GCSF). Bifunctional antibodies are currently constructed chemically by linking Fab preparations of each monoclonal with linkers such as o-phenylenedimaleimide (OPDM). It will be difficult to manufacture such products on a very large scale to meet market needs. Alternative methods through genetic engineering are likely to be developed.

Chimeric antibody C2B8 (anti-CD20) was examined in a phase I trial in 15 patients with low grade B cell lymphomas at doses of 10-500 mg/m^2. Serum half lives of 2-10 days were reported with tumor regression occurring in 6/15 patients. These responses are similar to that reported with radiolabeled anti-CD20 murine monoclonal antibodies and support the ability of human effector functions to mediate tumor clearance.[54]

Toxin-Monoclonal Antibody Conjugates

A number of trials with drug/toxin conjugates have been carried out (Table 4.4). The most extensively used toxins are the ricin A chain, *Pseudomonas* exotoxin A, diphtheria toxin, saporin and pokeweed antiviral protein.[73,74] Extensive developmental work has been carried out with monoclonal antibody-ricin conjugates. Early clinical studies produced a composite of symptoms thought to be generic to ricin A chain immunotoxins and most patients developed antibodies against the ricin A chain as well as a HAMA response.[58] The new generation of ricin based immunotoxins using deglycosylated forms of ricin A chain have shown only temporary toxicity. One, based upon anti-CD22-ricin showed a 60% mixed or partial response in 18 patients with refractory B cell leukemia/lymphoma.[64] Generally, responses achieving partial or complete remissions in lymphomas have been excellent (12-75%) particularly in comparison with prescribed drug response rates of around 5%.[73]

Table 4.4. Clinical trials with monoclonal - toxin conjugates

Antibody	Tumor	HAMA/TA (%)	Clinical response (%)	Reference
Ricin Conjugates:				
Xomazyme-791	colon	100	0	58
Xomazyme-Mel	melanoma	100	25	59
anti-CD19 (B4)	NHL	35-60	15	60-62
anti-CD22	NHL	35-50	25	63,64
anti-CD5	TCL/GVHD	75	20-50	65-67
260F9	breast	100	0	68,69
Saporin toxin:				
anti-CD30	Hodgkin's	100	75	70
Pseudomonas toxin:				
OVb3-PE	ovary	-	0	71
B3-PE38	breast	-	-	72

The common toxic symptoms are hepatotoxicity, vascular leak syndrome, myalgias and neutropenias.[73] Immune responses to both the antibody (HAMA) and toxin (HATA) are almost universal (Table 4.4) despite continual improvements in chemical conjugation techniques. To circumvent these problems, toxins of human origin are being investigated in the form of enzymes such as DNases, RNases, proteases and oxidoreductases[75] with promising in vivo data.[76]

DRUG-MONOCLONAL ANTIBODY CONJUGATES

The amount of toxin which can be delivered when fused to a monoclonal antibody is limited. Hence, it was felt necessary to use the very potent plant/microbial toxins but their side effects seriously limit dose levels. An exciting recent development has been the coupling of new highly potent synthetic chemotherapeutics such as adriamycin, aminopterin and calicheamicin to monoclonal antibodies.[77-80] Calicheamicin conjugates have been shown to have potent anti-tumor activity in vivo in animal models.[80] A chimeric BR96 monoclonal antibody, with specificity for Lewis Y antigen, conjugated to doxorubicin has been shown, in trials by Bristol-Myers Squibb, to achieve 70% clearance of tumors and 80% survival in mice. It is hoped that these small organics with a molecular weight of approximately 1500 Da will not induce an antibody response.

ENZYME-MONOCLONAL ANTIBODY CONJUGATES

Antibody directed enzyme pro-drug therapy (ADEPT) is a two stage procedure where pro-drugs are converted to active drug at the site of the tumor by means of previously delivered antibody-enzyme conjugates.[81] Enzymes which have been linked to monoclonal antibodies include carboxypeptidase, alkaline phosphatase, glucuronidase and β-lactamase and recently, single chain antibody fragments fused to β-lactamase and alkaline phosphatase have been produced by recombinant DNA technology.[82,83]

RADIOLABELED MONOCLONAL ANTIBODIES IN THERAPY

^{131}I, the radioisotope most commonly used in the past for therapy, is being replaced by ^{90}Y or ^{188}Re as the conjugate of choice. Trials involving a number of radiolabeled antibodies are in progress (Table 4.5). The main difficulties remain low radioactive uptake by the tumor, bone marrow toxicity, heterogeneity of tumor cells and HAMA response. Better results are achieved against lymphomas and leukemias than with solid tumors. The importance of achieving increased radioactive uptake is exemplified by recent preclinical animal studies with a cocktail of three ^{131}I labeled $F(ab')_2$ fragments against different CEA epitopes. Complete tumor remission was observed in 14 nude mice with colorectal tumor xenografts.[101] Radiation doses greater than 80 Gy were delivered to the tumor by the cocktail [1 gray (Gy) = 100 rad = 1 J/kg].

Early trials with ^{131}I labeled monoclonal antibody HMFG2 in a number of clinical studies showed that products could be used with minimal toxicity and some partial or complete remissions were recorded.[91] Fifty two patients with ovarian cancer were treated with ^{90}Y-labeled HMFG1 following conventional surgery and chemotherapy.[90] A five year follow up has shown significantly improved survival rates and extended remissions. Responses of leukemias and lymphomas have also been hopeful, particularly when monoclonal antibody treatment was followed by autologous marrow rescue to overcome myleosuppression which is observed in all patients. Extended remissions have been reported.[1,86,87] Results with monoclonal antibody B1 which has a specificity for CD20 have been particu-

Table 4.5. Immunotherapy trials with radiolabeled monoclonal antibodies

Antibody	Antigen	Tumor	HAMA (%)	Reference
^{131}I-B72.3	TAG-72	colon	58-75	84,85
^{131}I-B1	CD20	lymphoma	22-33	86,87
^{131}I-CC49	TAG-72	colon	100	88
^{90}Y-B72.3	TAG-72	ovary	-	89
^{90}Y-HMFG1	mucin	ovary	-	90
^{131}I-HMFG2	mucin	-	-	91
^{186}Re-LU-10	-	ovary	-	92
^{131}I-Lym-1	HLA-Dr	CLL	20	93
^{90}Y-anti ferritin	ferritin	lymphoma	-	94
^{131}I-OKB7	CD21	NHL	75	95
^{131}I-MB-1	-	B cell lymphoma	-	1
^{131}I-M195	CD33	AML	37	96
^{90}Y-T101	CD5	B/T malignancies	-	1
^{131}I-LL2	-	B cell lymphoma	-	97
^{131}I-anti CEA	CEA	thyroid	-	98
^{131}I-A5B7	CEA	colon	-	99
^{131}I-L6	-	breast	24	100

larly encouraging. The overall response rate in 19 patients with lymphomas refractory to chemotherapy was 84% and complete remission occurred in 50%.[87] It is likely that this good response was due to a combination of radiation lethality and cell killing due the monoclonal antibody itself through ADCC.

Myelosuppression is also reduced by repetitive administration of multiple fractionated non-myeloabalative doses rather than a single massive dose. Fractionated therapy with ^{131}I labeled Lym-1, an IgG_{2a}, resulted in an overall response rate of about 60% in refractory non-Hodgkin's lymphoma patients with advanced disease.[93] A clinical trial using ^{67}Cu labeled Lym-1 against non-Hodgkin's lymphoma is now in progress.

A ^{90}Y-B72.3 phase I trial in 40 patients with ovarian cancer showed only two remissions but demonstrated that the haematological toxicity and bone accumulation by this radionuclide could be reduced effectively by combination treatment with the chelating agent EDTA. This has the effect of accelerating urinary excretion.[89] Over 100 patients with hepatoma have been treated with ^{131}I or ^{90}Y labeled anti-ferritin.[94] Up to a 48% response was observed with 7% showing complete remission. ^{90}Y-anti-ferritin monoclonal antibodies have been used to treat ferritin rich lymphomas in patients with recurrent Hodgkin's disease and some response noted.

Anti-Carcinoembryonic (CEA) Monoclonal Antibodies

Anti-CEA monoclonal antibodies are one of the most widely studied. The Immunomedics product (ImmuRAID-CEA: IMMU-4) as an Fab labeled with Tc99m failed to gain FDA approval for colorectal imaging in May 1994 but is in phase III trials for lung cancer imaging and phase II trials for breast cancer imaging. In a multi-center phase II trial of 54 patients with diverse lung cancers, the overall sensitivity of detection was 90% and the accuracy was 85%.

In earlier phase I studies, less than 1% of patients showed a HAMA response. A different anti-CEA, A537 has been used in patients with advanced CEA-positive tumors[99] and concomitant dosing with cyclosporine A extended the length of treatment to four doses in 60 days before a HAMA response appeared. A Rhenium-labeled derivative is in phase I/II clinical trials for the treatment of colorectal cancer and a humanized version has now been developed. The alternate Cytogen product, Oncoscint CEA, is currently in Phase I trials.

B72.3 (ONCOSCINT CR/OV) is a murine IgG with specificity for an oncofetal antigen termed TAG-72 (sialyl-Tn) and is reactive with a broad range of carcinomas including colorectal, gastric, pancreatic, ovarian, endometrial, prostate and non-small cell lung. This was the first monoclonal antibody based imaging agent to be approved by the FDA (in December 1992) for the detection of metastatic colorectal cancer and metastatic ovarian cancer to be used in combination with computer aided tomography (CT) scanning. In a two year study comparing chest X-ray, colonoscopy and CT imaging with ^{111}In labeled B72.3, the rate of detection of occult colorectal cancer recurrence was 91.6% compared to 20.6% detection rate of CT: colonoscopy and chest X-ray remained negative during the 12 month study period. In imaging ovarian cancer,[22] the antibody correctly detected the presence and extent of residual disease in 83% of patients with residual neoplasia at laparotomy compared with 50% detected by CT and 75% by serum CA125 assays. In such studies, a HAMA response occurs in about 23% of patients.

A novel use for ^{125}I-labeled B72.3 has been the detection of occult tumors and breast carcinomas using a hand-held ^{90}Y detecting probe.[26,102] This approach, termed radioimmunoguided surgery (RIGS) is being pursued by Neoprobe Inc. More effective surgery was carried out thereafter since residual and subclinical sites were detected. Clinical studies with B72.3 have been summarized recently.[5] ^{131}I labeled chimeric B72.3 has been used in phase I trials in metastatic colon cancer but no responses were recorded in 12 patients.[84,85] Seven out of twelve patients developed a HAMA response which is similar to that recorded for the mouse implying the variable region to be the principal immunogenic component of this antibody. ^{90}Y labeled B72.3 (OncoRad OV103) is in phase II for the treatment of ovarian cancer.[89] A humanized version of this antibody is now available.

CC49 is a second generation B72.3 monoclonal antibody raised by immunizing mice with antigen purified using B72.3. It has about an 8-fold higher affinity than B72.3 and binds to a range of carcinomas including colorectal, gastric, pancreatic, ovarian, mammary, lung and prostate. In a phase I trial treating metastatic colon cancer, only 1 patient of 24 showed a minor response and all developed a HAMA response.[88] A phase III trial is in progress using ^{131}I labeled CC49. This antibody has also been licensed to Neoprobe Inc. for use in RIGS technology. A humanized version of CC49 is being developed.

Murine 17-1A, an IgG_{2a} has been one of the most studied monoclonal antibodies since it was produced in 1978. It binds to a tumor associated 37 kDa glycoprotein antigen. 17-1A, even at radiolabeled doses as low as 0.1 mg, efficiently localizes metastatic lesions on colorectal cancer[103] and gram quantities of 17-1A have been administered to patients with no evidence of toxicity.[104] Six clinical studies have been carried out in metastatic colorectal patients with murine 17-1A.[6] The serum half life averages 16-30 hours with a HAMA response of between 50 and 100% in the various studies. Only sporadic clinical responses have been noted.

Mouse-human chimeric antibodies for all human IgG subclasses and IgM have been constructed. The IgG_1, κ chimeric formulation was the first chimeric antibody to be taken into clinical trial. Serum half life is increased 5-8-fold over the murine version to average 100 hours and immune response was noted in only 2/32 patients. This reduction in immune response contrasts with the more modest reduction recorded with chimeric B72.3 suggesting that the immunogenicity of murine variable regions may vary dramatically.

Monoclonal antibody M195 recognizes CD33. Imaging studies showed that ^{131}I-M195 effectively targeted leukemic cells with bone marrow imaging stable for up to three days after infusion.[105] This stability of binding greatly increases therapeutic potential. Twelve patients with relapsed or refractory myeloid malignancies were treated with ^{131}I-M195 before bone marrow transplant (BMT).[96] After 10 months follow-up, seven were alive and six had been in remission for 4-25 months. Thirty seven percent of patients developed a HAMA response thereby preventing further treatment. A humanized version of this antibody has been developed and clinical trials are underway.

Autoimmune Disease

Monoclonal antibodies are under evaluation for the treatment of most autoimmune diseases with the ultimate aim of selective depletion of the patients pathogenic T and B cell populations (Table 4.6). Since chronic administration is likely to be required many promising murine antibodies are being humanized prior to clinical trials. The use of monoclonal antibodies to modulate immune responses has been reviewed recently.[116] Targets include complete elimination of T cells or specific T cells subsets, blocking of adhesion receptors on T cells to achieve temporary immunosuppression or long term tolerance and the specific elimination of B cell populations which recognize self antigens.

TRANSPLANTATION

Ex vivo use of monoclonal antibodies

Research over many years has repeatedly confirmed that organ rejection after transplantation in animal studies can arise from the transfer of immunogenic passenger cells along with the organ. Thus, in vitro culture of organs prior to transplantation reduces rejection as does pre-treatment with HLA class II specific antibodies.[117] Antibodies have now been used successfully to reduce frequencies of rejection by pre-treatment of human donor organs. A pair of complement-lytic synergistic anti-CD45 antibodies with reactivity against dendritic cells, when infused into donor organs, significantly reduces rejection episodes.[118]

Two milligrams each of rat anti-CD45 monoclonal antibodies YTH 24.5 and YTH 54.12 were perfused into kidneys prior to transplant and 40 patients were observed over a three month period. No adverse clinical effects were noted though two patients developed an anti-rat antibody response. Where antibody uptake

Table 4.6. Monoclonal antibodies in clinical trial for immunosuppression and immunomodulation in transplantation and autoimmunity

Antibody	Antigen	Effect	Reference
CAMPATH-1	mononuclear	non-specific	109
OKT-3	CD3	all T cells	106
anti-CD4	T-helper	tolerance	108
anti-CD54	ICAM-1 (CD54)	adhesion inhibition	110
anti-CD25:			
33B3.1	IL-2 receptor (CD25)	activated T cells only	111
anti-Tac	IL-2 receptor (CD25)	activated T cells only	112
CAMPATH-6	IL-2 receptor (CD25)	activated T cells only	113
anti-CD7	CD7	all T cells	114
cA2	TNFα	activated T cells only	115

into the donor kidney was high, a rejection rate of 18% was noted compared with a rejection rate of 63% in controls. A larger scale placebo-controlled trial is now ongoing

Orthoclone OKT3 is the most common antibody used in transplantation and is directed against the CD3 component of cell surface T cell receptor complexes. Given intravenously, OKT3 causes rapid removal of $CD3^+$ T cells from the circulation and thereby prevents killing by cytotoxic T cells. Many T cells modulate their cell surface expression after binding OKT3 and the peripheral blood is then replenished after cessation of treatment. It's primary use has been as an immunosuppressive agent and its efficacy in reducing rejection during renal transplant is well established.[106] OKT3 has been approved for this application since 1986. Typical therapy is 5 mg/day intravenously for 10-14 days. Ninety percent of US transplant centers use OKT3 for prophylaxis against renal allograft rejection and about 50% of US centers use it for cardiac and hepatic transplants. Two year graft survival rates are higher where OKT3 is used prophylactically (84%) compared with cyclosporine alone (75%).[107]

The limitations to therapy arise from the HAMA responses from prolonged or repeat infusion, cytokine release syndrome and increased susceptibility to infection due to general immunosuppression. OKT3 is not successful in bone marrow transplants[119] but it may prove useful in the future for human islet transplants.[117] A humanized version of this antibody had been developed.

Murine OKT4a recognizes CD4 and can be used to deplete $CD4^+$ or helper T cells. These cells recognize antigen usually concomitantly with class II MHC and secrete cytokines that promote B cell antibody responses to the inducing antigen. Anti-CD4 monoclonal antibodies can therefore be used to induce tolerance to murine monoclonal antibodies, and a number of different anti-CD4 monoclonal antibodies have been tried in autoimmune or transplant indications.[108] OKT4a has been given as a single dose to cardiac transplant patients but CD4 receptors were not saturated and HAMA was induced. Treatment has also been given to patients with rheumatoid arthritis with similar results. A multiple dose regime (0.2 mg/kg/day for 8-12 days) was given to six patients for renal prophylaxis. Serum levels of OKT4a reduced rapidly, antibody was undetectable after 24 hours and 100% of the patients developed a HAMA response. A humanized version of the antibody is now available and further clinical studies will be with this product.

CAMPATH-1M is a rat IgM monoclonal antibody identified from a group of monoclonal antibodies which were unusually lytic for human lymphocytes. All of these antibodies were reactive with a small glycoprotein attached to the cell membrane by the GP 1 anchor, the antigen being designated CAMPATH-1 (CDw52).[109] Since 1983, more than 500 transplants have been performed in 23 transplant centers in Europe using CAMPATH-1M for T cell depletion. The incidence of severe or chronic graft-versus-host-disease (GVHD) is significantly reduced. The frequency of acute GVHD (grade 1) in patients at risk was 17% and only 7% in severe acute GVHD (grade 3-4). The frequency of chronic GVHD was 19% and severe chronic GVHD only 2%.[120]

CAMPATH-1G is a rat IgG_{2b} antibody reactive against CDw52 and is very efficient at depleting lymphocytes since the rat IgG_{2b} subclass is the most potent for activating human complement and for binding to human Fc receptors. Studies involving 75 patients with acute leukemia in first remission have been carried out with promising results. Only 2% showed severe acute GVHD. There were no cases of severe chronic GVHD and only 9% graft failure. Mortality at two years from all causes other than relapse was significantly reduced and leukemia free survival is much better.[120]

CAMPATH-1M and -1G have also been used successfully in transplantation for non-malignant diseases, aplastic anemia, thallasemias and Fanconi's anemia. One hundred and sixteen such transplants have been carried out using a mixture of protocols with T cell depletion of donor organs in vitro prior to transplant along with in vivo treatment of recipients.[120] A humanized version of CAMPATH-1G is now available and data are discussed in chapter 6.

CD7 and CD25 are two cell surface antigens whose expression is upgraded after stimulation by antigen. Monoclonal antibodies RFT2 (anti-CD7) and RFT5 (anti-CD25) are murine IgG_{2a} monoclonals developed by Sandoz and have been converted into IgG1/κ murine-human chimeric antibodies described as SDZ CHH380 (anti-CD7) and SDZ CHI621 (anti-CD25) respectively. CHH380 has been studied in phase I clinical trials in renal transplant and rheumatoid arthritis patients and in phase II/III trials in rheumatoid arthritis. Side effects included flu-like symptoms and diarrhea but were mild compared with OKT3 and lasted only a few hours. The serum half life was 2-5 days compared to 1 day with the parental murine monoclonal antibody. Since CD7 antigen is expressed on most T cells the short half life is partially attributable to adsorption to T cells in tissues. Only 1/115 patients displayed a HAMA response. Improvement upon frequency of rejection in renal transplant patients was seen though the data were not statistically significant.[114]

No adverse clinical effects were noted in a phase I trial in renal transplant patients with CHI621 and the serum half-life was 13 days, which approaches the 21 days expected for human IgG_1. No HAMA was found in the 24 patients treated and some reduction in the number of rejection episodes was noted. A multicenter phase III trial is ongoing. Three anti-CD25 monoclonal antibodies have been evaluated. 33B3.1 (rat IgG_{2a}), when given along with prednisone and azathioprine, prevented early rejection during renal transplant and a 2 year follow-up showed that antibody treated patients had fewer infection episodes, especially urinary infections.[111] A reduction in rejection was also noted with anti-Tac (murine IgG_{2a}) during renal transplantation[112] and CAMPATH-6 (rat IgG_{2b}) during liver transplants.[113] Both 33B3.1 and anti-Tac recognize the α-chain (p55: Tac antigen) of the IL-2 receptor but show different behavior in biological assays. It seems that orientation of antigen-antibody may be crucial for clinical effectiveness. Anti-Tac has been humanized and taken into trial.

Systemic Lupus Erythromatosus

In the case of systemic lupus erythromatosus (SLE), autoantibodies to DNA play a major role in disease pathogenesis and efforts have focused upon inducing the development of anti-idiotypic antibodies to shared cross reactive epitopes in patients, anti-DNA sera. Monoclonal antibody 3E10 (MedClone Inc.), a murine antibody with specificity for human kidney, has completed a six patient phase I trial for the treatment of SLE with the antibody being described as safe and efficacious in provoking an anti-idiotypic response, suggesting a role for the antibody as a therapeutic vaccine.

Rheumatoid Arthritis

Adhesion molecules which mediate intercellular interactions, such as occur during the recruitment of inflammatory cells to sites of damage, are the targets for a broad range of antibody based therapies.[121] In particular, leukocyte-function associated antigen-1 (LFA-1: CD11a/CD18) and intercellular adhesion molecule-1 (ICAM-1; CD54) play a central role in the migration of T lymphocytes. They are, therefore, attractive targets for T cell mediated diseases and a number of monoclonal antibodies against these antigens have been humanized.

A mouse-human chimeric antibody cA2 (Centocor) against TNFα has been used in a preliminary trial in rheumatoid arthritis patients.[115] During the course of treatment, 16 patients showed measurable clinical benefit in subjective and objective parameters such as swollen and tender joint scores, morning stiffness and locomotor functions but the disease reappeared several weeks after cessation of treatment. Similar results have been obtained with anti-CD4 and CAMPATH-1H.

R6.5 (BIRR1), a murine IgG_{2a} against ICAM-1 (CD54) has been evaluated in a phase I study in rheumatoid arthritis patients refractory to conventional therapy.[110] Twenty-three patients received doses of up to 560 mg over a five day period and 13/23 showed a marked or moderate response to symptoms such as tender or swollen joints, duration of morning stiffness etc., for up to 29 days, with 9/23 still showing improvement at day 60. All the patients developed a HAMA response by day 15. Some patients sustained clinical efficacy for several months but all eventually reverted. Nevertheless this study provides encouragement that a short duration of treatment which interferes with the recirculation of T lymphocytes may have extended clinical effects. Humanized anti-ICAM-1 monoclonal antibodies devoid of HAMA may provide a basis for chronic treatment.[110]

Cardiovascular

Monoclonal antibody 7E3 (Centocor) recognizes the integrin IIb/IIIa receptor on the surface of platelets and prevents platelet aggregation by blocking the binding of circulating adhesive factors such as fibrinogen and von Willebrand factor. The antibody has been shown to have anti thrombotic effects in animal models, and in a phase I study it inhibited platelet aggregation by more than 80% in patients undergoing coronary angioplasty.[122] The antibody was genetically engineered as a mouse-human chimeric (murine VH/VL: Human CIgG) and the Fab fragment used in a study in high risk coronary angioplasty.[123] An initial trial showed that inhibition of platelet aggregation was beneficial in preventing abrupt vessel closure by a thrombus at the site of angioplasty and supports the concept that inhibition of platelet interactions is a way to prevent acute complications after coronary angioplasty or atherectomy. However, to achieve this benefit it is necessary to block almost all the IIb/IIIa epitopes on circulating platelets and this resulted in an excess of bleeding events. A large trial with 2099 patients has confirmed this general conclusion. At six months, there was a 23% reduction in ischemic events (death, nonfatal myocardial infarction (MI), need for revascularization) and a 26% decrease in target vessel revascularization.[122] However, the side effects of excess bleeding and need for transfusions will need to be overcome before wider use.

CONCLUSIONS

Considering the almost universal HAMA response in patients the data discussed above is encouraging. Cancer is a very difficult target for any form of therapy and yet some efficacy has been shown for rodent and chimeric monoclonals in lymphomas and leukemias. Poor access of intact antibody to solid tumors is likely to be a major factor in poor clinical responses here but future use of antibody fragments may provide a partial solution to this problem.

Immunosuppression through monoclonal antibodies has been successful in solid organ transplants and some temporary clinical value has been obtained in reducing the symptoms of rheumatoid arthritis through inhibition of CD4 and adhesion factors.

Many of the antibodies described in this chapter have now been humanized and offer good prospects for future therapy.

REFERENCES

1. Broder S ed. Molecular and Cellular Research for Future Diagnosis and Therapy. Baltimore: Williams and Wilkins, 1990.
2. Reynolds JC, Del Vecchio S, Sakahara H et al. Anti-murine response to mouse monoclonal antibodies: clinical findings and implications. Nucl Med Biol 1989; 16:121-125.
3. Morrison SL, Oi VT. Genetically engineered antibody molecules. Adv Immunol 1989; 44:65-91.
4. Adair JR. Engineering antibodies for therapy. Immunol Rev 1992; 130:5-40.
5. Adair JR, Baker TS, Bebbington CR et al. Engineering monoclonal antibody B72.3 for cancer therapy. In: Clark M ed. Protein Engi-

neering of Antibody Molecules for Prophylaxis and Therapeutic Applications in Man. Nottingham: Academic Press, 1993:145-158.

6. LoBuglio AF, Khazaeli MB. Clinical studies with murine and chimeric 17-1A in colorectal cancer patients. In: Clark M ed. Protein Engineering of Antibody Molecules for Prophylaxis and Therapeutic Applications in Man. Nottingham: Academic Press, 1993:171-177.
7. Zuckier LS, Rodriguez LD, Scharff MD. Immunologic and pharmacologic concepts of monoclonal antibodies. Sem Nucl Med 1989; 19:166-186.
8. Colcher D, Bird R, Roselli M et al. *In vivo* tumour targetting of a recombinant single-chain antigen-binding protein. J Natl Cancer Inst 1990; 82:1191-1197.
9. Wood DM, Parent JB, Gazzano-Santori H et al. Reactivity of monoclonal antibody E5 with endotoxin; 1. binding to lipid A and rough lipopolysaccharides. Circulatory Shock 1992; 38:55-62.
10. Parent JB, Gazzano-Santori H, Wood DM et al. Reactivity of monoclonal antibody E5-11 binding to short and long chain smooth lipopolysaccharides. Cirulatory Shock 1992; 38:63-73.
11. Greenman RL, Schein RM, Martin MA et al. A controlled clinical trial of E5 murine monoclonal IgM antibody to endotoxin in the treatment of gram negative sepsis. J Am Med Assoc 1991; 266:1097-1102.
12. D'Souza MP, Geyer SJ, Hanson CV et al. Evaluation of monoclonal antibodies to HIV-1 envelope by neutralisation and binding assays: an international collaboration. AIDS 1994; 8:169-181.
13. Loveless MD. Early clinical trials of anti-HIV antibodies in AIDS: What lessons can we learn. Antibody Based Therapeutics: the latest Clinical Trial and Applications Strategies BC Conference, Washington, June 1994.
14. Mach JP, Chatal JF, Lumbroso JD et al. Tumour localisation in patients by radiolabelled monoclonal antibodies against colon carcinoma. Cancer Res 1983; 43:5593-5600.
15. Goldenberg DM, Kimm EE, Bennett SJ et al. Carcinembryonic antigen radioimmunodetection in the evaluation of colorectal cancer in the detection of occult neoplasms. Gastroenterology 1983; 84:524-532.
16. Siccardi AG, Buraggi GL, Callegaro L et al. Immunoscintigraphy of adenocarcinomas by means of radiolabeled $F(ab')_2$ fragments of an anti-carcinoembryonic antigen monoclonal antibody: a multicenter study. Cancer Res 1989; 49:3095-3103.
17. Krishnamurthy S, Morris JF, Antanovic R et al. Evaluation of primary lung cancer with indium-111 anti-carcinoembryonic antigen (type ZCE-025) monoclonal antibody scintigraphy. Cancer 1990; 65:458-465.
18. Esteban JM, Colcher D, Sugarbaker P et al. Quantitative and qualitative aspects of radiolocalisation in colon cancer patients of intra-

venous administered mAb 72.3. Int J Cancer 1987; 39:50-59.
19. Renda A, Salvatore M, Sava M et al. Immunoscintigraphy in the follow-up of patients operated on for carcinoma of the sigmoid and rectum. Dis Colon Rectum 1987; 30:683-686.
20. Maguire TR, Schmelter RF, Pascucci VL et al. Immunoscintigraphy of colorectal adenocarcinoma: results with site-specifically radiolabelled B72.3 (^{111}In-CYT-103). Antibod Immunoconj Radiopharm 1989; 2:257-269.
21. Lastoria S, D'Amico P, Manis L et al. A prospective imaging study of ^{131}1-B72.3 monoclonal antibody in patients with epithelial ovarian cancer. Preliminary Report. Nucl Med Com 1988; 9:347-356.
22. Neal CE, Baker MR, Hilgers RD et al. In-111 CYT-103 immunoscintigraphy in the imaging of ovarian cancer. Clin Nucl Med 1993; 18;472-476.
23. Anonymous. Update: radioimmunoconjugates in cancer diagnosis and therapy. Drug and Market Development 1994; 5:38-44.
24. Goldenberg DM, Schlom J. The coming of age of radioimmunoconjugates. Immunology Today 1993; 14:5-7.
25. Moldofsky PJ, Powe J, Mulhern CB et al. Metastatic colon carcinoma detected with radiolabelled F(ab')$_2$ monoclonal antibody fragments. Radiology 1983; 149:549-555.
26. Nieroda CA, Mojzisik C, Sardi A et al. Staging of carcinoma of the breast using a hand held gamma detecting probe and monoclonal antibody B72.3. Surg Gynecol Obstet 1989; 169:35-40
27. Bast RC, Freeney M, Lazarus H et al. Reactivity of a monoclonal antibody with human ovarian carcinoma. J Clin Invest 1981; 68:1331-1337.
28. Eppenitos AA, Munro AJ, Stewart S et al. Antibody guided irradiation of advanced ovarian cancer with intraperitoneally administered monoclonal antibodies. J Clin Oncol 1987; 5:1890-1899.
29. Pectasides D, Stewart S, Courtenay-Luck N et al. Antibody guided irradiation of malignant pleural and perocardial effusions. Br J Cancer 1986; 53:727-732.
30. Larson SM, Carrasquillo JA, Krohn KA et al. Localisation of ^{131}I labelled p97 specific Fab fragments in human melanoma as a basis for radiotherapy. J Clin Invest 1983; 72:2101-2114.
31. DeNardo SJ, DeNardo GL, O'Grady LF et al. Treatment of B cell malignancies with ^{131}I lym-1 monoclonal antibodies. Int J Cancer (Suppl) 1988; 3:96-101.
32. Salk D. Technetium labelled monoclonal antibodies for imaging metastatic melanoma; results of a multicenter clinical study. Semin Oncol 1988; 15:608-618.
33. Bander NH. Monoclonal antibodies to renal cancer antigens. Eur Urol (suppl) 1990; 18:2-10.
34. Jain D, Lahiri A, Raftery EB. Immunoscintigraphy for detecting acute myocardial infarction without electrocadiographic changes. Brit Med J 1990; 300:151-153.

35. Nadler LM, Stashenko P, Hardy R et al. Serotherapy of a patient with a monoclonal antibody directed against a human lymphoma associated antigen. Cancer Res 1980; 40:3147-3154.
36. Ritz J, Pesando JM, Sallan SE et al. Serotherapy of acute lymphoblastic leukemia with monoclonal antibody. Blood 1981; 58: 141-152.
37. Mellstedt H, Frodin J-E, Masucci G et al. The therapeutic use of monoclonal antibodies in colorectal carcinoma. Sem Oncol 1991; 18:462-477.
38. Houghton AN, Mintzer D, Cordon-Cardo C et al. Mouse monoclonal IgG_3 antibody detecting GD3 ganglioside: A phase I trial in patients with malignant melanoma.
39. Traub UC, DeJager RL, Primus FJ et al. Anti-idiotype antibodies in cancer patients receiving monoclonal antibody to carcino-embryonic antigen. Cancer Res 1988; 48:4002-4006.
40. Raubitschek A, Colcher D, Lastoria S et al. Intraperitoneally administered radiolabeled monoclonal antibodies in patients with peritoneal carcinomatosis. (Abstract) Second Conference on Radioimmunodetection and Radioimmunotherapy of Cancer, Princeton NJ, 1988.
41. Cheung NK, Lazarus H, Miraldi FD et al. Ganglioside GD2 specific monoclonal antibody 3F8: a phase I study in patients with neuroblastoma and malignant melanoma. J Clin Oncol 1987; 5:1430-1440.
42. Goodman GE, Beaumier P, Hellstrom I et al. Pilot trial of murine monoclonal antibodies in patients with advanced melanoma. J Clin Oncol 1985; 3:340-352.
43. Dillman RO, Beauregard J, Shawler DL et al. Continuous infusion of T101 monoclonal antibody in chronic lymphocytic leukemia and cutaneous T cell lymphoma. J Biol Res Mod 1986; 3:394-410.
44. Miller RA, Maloney DG, McKillop J et al. In vivo effects of murine hybridoma monoclonal antibody in patients with T cell leukemia. Blood 1981; 58:78-86.
45. Fanger MW. Bispecific Antibodies. Austin: RG Landes Co, 1995.
46. Waldmann TA, Goldman CK, Bongiovanni KF et al. Therapy of patients with human T-cell lymphotropic virus induced adult T cell leukemia with anti-tac, a monoclonal to the receptor for interleukin-2. Blood 1988; 72:1805-1816.
47. Dyer MJS, Hale G, Hayhoe FGJ et al. Effects of CAMPATH-1 antibodies *in vivo* in patients with lymphoid malignancies: Influence of antibody isotype. Blood 1989; 73:1431-1439.
48. Goodman GE, Hellstrom I, Brodzinsky L et al. Phase I trial of murine monoclonal antibody L6 in breast colon ovarian and lung cancer. J Clin Oncol 1990; 8:1083-1092.
49. Weiner LMW. Bispecific monoclonal antibody therapy. Proc IBC Conference: Antibody Based Therapeutics; Washington, 1994.
50. Bolhuis RLH, Lamers CHJ, Goey SH et al. Adoptive immunotherapy of ovarian carcinoma with BS-Mab-targeted lymphocytes: a multicenter study. Int J Cancer 1992; 7:78-81.

51. Valone FH. Clinical trials of bispecific antibody MDX-210 (anti-her-2/neu x anti-FcR1(CD64)) for treatment of breast and ovarian cancer. Proc IBC Conference: Antibody Engineering; La Jolla, 1994.
52. Meredith RF, Khazaeli MB, Plott WE et al. Comparison of two mouse/human chimeric antibodies in patients with metastatic colon cancer. Antibod Immunoconj Radiopharm 1992; 5:75-80.
53. Lo Buglio AF, Wheeler RH, Trang J et al. Mouse/human chimeric monoclonal antibody in man: kinetics and immune reponse. Proc Nat Acad Sci 1989; 86:4220-4224.
54. Grillo-Lopez AJ, Rosenberg J, McClure A et al. Early clinical trials with a monoclonal anti-CD20 antibody. IBC cnf: Antibody Based Therapeutics, Washington, 1994.
55. Miller RA, Maloney DG, Warnke R et al. Treatment of B cell lymphoma with monoclonal anti-idioytpe antibody. N Eng J Med 1982; 306:517-522.
56. Meeker TC, Lowder J, Maloney DG et al. A clinical trial of anti-Id therapy for B cell malignancy. Blood 1985; 656:1359-1363.
57. Miller RA, Hart S, Samoszuk M et al. Shared idiotypes expressed by human B cell lymphomas. N Eng J Med 1989; 321:851-857.
58. Byers VS, Rodvein R, Grant K et al. Phase I study of monoclonal antibody ricin A chain immunotoxin XomaZyme-791 in patients with metastatic colon cancer. Cancer Res 1989; 49:6153-6160.
59. Selvaggi K, Saria EA, Schwartz R et al. Phase I/II study of murine monoclonal antibody-ricin A chain (Xomazyme-mel) immunoconjugate plus cyclosporine A in patients with metastatic melanoma. J Immunother 1993; 13:201-207.
60. Grossbard ML, Freedman AS, Ritz J et al. Serotherapy of B cell neoplasms with anti-B4 blocked ricin: a phase I trial of daily bolus infusion. Blood 1992; 79:576-585.
61. Grossbard ML, Lambert JM, Goldmacher VS et al. Anti-B-4 blocked ricin; a phase I trial of 7-day continous infusion in patients with B cell neoplasms. J Clin Oncol 1993; 11:726-737.
62. Grossbard ML, Gribben JG, Freedman AS et al. Adjuvant immunotoxin therapy with anti-B4 blocked ricin after autologous bone marrow transplantation for patients with B cell non-Hodgkin's lymphoma. Blood 1993; 81:2263-2271.
63. Vitetta ES, Stone M, Amlot P et al. Phase I immunotoxin trial in patients with B cell lymphoma. Cancer Res 1991; 51:4052-4058.
64. Amlot PL, Stone MJ, Cunningham D et al. A phase I study of an anti-CD22 deglycosylated ricin A chain immunotoxin in the treatment of B cell lymphomas resistant to conventional therapy. Blood 1993: 82:2624-2633.
65. LeMaistre CF, Rosen F, Frankel A et al. Phase I trial of H65-RTA immunoconjugate in patients with cutaneous T-cell lymphoma. Blood 1991; 78:1173-1182.
66. Weisdorf D, Filipovitch A, McGlave P et al. Combination graft-versus-host disease prophylaxis using immunotoxin (anti-CD5-RTA

[Xomazyme-CD5]) plus methotrexate and cyclosporine or prednisone after unrelated bone marrow transplantation. Bone Marrow Transplant 1993; 12:531-536.
67. Byers VS, Henslee PJ, Kernan NA et al. Use of anti-pan T-lymphocyte ricin A chain immunotoxin in steroid-resistant acute graft-versus-host disease. Blood 1990; 75:1426-1432.
68. Weiner LM, O'Dwyer J, Kitson J et al. Phase I evaluation of an anti-breast carcinoma monoclonal antibody 260F9-recombinant ricin A chain immunoconjugate. Cancer Res 1989; 49:4062-4067.
69. Gould BJ, Borowitz MJ, Groves ES et al. Phase I study of an anti-breast cancer immunotoxin by continous infusion: report of a targeted toxic effect not predicted by animal studies. J Natl Cancer Inst 1989; 81:775-781.
70. Falini B, Bolognesi A, Flenghi L et al. Response of refractory Hodgkin's disease to monoclonal anti-CD30-immunotoxin. Lancet 1992; 339:1195-1196.
71. Pai LH, Bookman MA, Ozols RF et al. Clinical evaluation of intraperitoneal Pseudomonas exotoxin immunoconjugate OVB3-PE in patients with ovarian cancer. J Clin Oncol 1991; 9:2095-2103.
72. Pai LH, Batra JK, FitGerald DJ et al. Anti-tumour effects of B3-PE and B3-lysPE40 in a nude mouse model of human breast cancer and the evaluation of B3-PE toxicity in monkeys. Cancer Res 1992; 52:3189-3193.
73. Vitetta ES, Thorpe PE, Uhr JW. Immunotoxins: magic bullets or misguided missiles? Immunology Today 1993; 14:252-259.
74. Pai LH, Pastan I. Immunotoxin Therapy for Cancer. JAMA 1993; 269:78-81.
75. Gadina M, Newton DL, Rybak SM et al. Humanized immunotoxins. Therap Immunol 1994; 1:59-64.
76. Newton DL, Ilercil O, Laske DW et al. Cytotoxic ribonuclease chimeras; targeted tumouricidal activity in vitro and in vivo. J Biol Chem 1992; 267:19572-19578.
77. Koppel GA. Recent advances with monoclonal antibody drug targeting for the treatment of human cancer. Bioconjugate Chem 1990; 1:13-23.
78. Chari RVJ, Martell BA, Gross JL et al. Immunoconjugates containing novel maytansinoids: promising anticancer drugs. Cancer Res 1992; 52:127-131.
79. Krauer KG, Bell R, Pietersz GA. Aminopterin-monoclonal antibody conjugates. Antitumour activity and toxicity. Drug Targeting Delivery 1993; 1:27-33.
80. Hinman LM, Hamann PR, Wallace R et al Preparation and characterisation of monoclonal antibody conjugates of the calicheamicins; a novel and potent family of antitumour antibiotics. Cancer Res 1993; 53:3336-3342.
81. Senter PD. Activation of prodrugs by antibody-enzyme conjugates: a new approach to cancer therapy. FASEB J 1990; 4:188-193.

82. Deonarain MP, Epenetos AA. Targeting enzymes for cancer therapy: old enzymes in new roles. Br J Cancer 1994; 70:786-794.
83. Goshorn SC, Svensson HP, Kerr DE et al. Genetic construction, expression and characterisation of a single-chain anti-carcinoma antibody fused to beta-lactamase. Cancer Res 1993; 53:2123-2127.
84. Meredith RF, Khazaeli MB, Plot WE et al. Phase I trial of iodine-131-chimeric B72.3 (Human IgG_4) in metastatic colorectal cancer. J Nuc Med 1992; 33:23-29.
85. Meredith RF, Khazaeli MB, Lui T et al. Dose fractionation of radiolabeled antibodies in patients with metastatic colon cancer. J Nuc Med 1992; 3:1648-1653.
86. Press OW, Eary JF, Appelbaum FR et al. Radiolabeled antibody therapy of B cell lymphoma with autologous bone marrow support. New Eng J Med 1993; 329:1219-1224.
87. Kaminski MS, Zasadny KR, Francis IR et al. Radioimmunotherapy of B cell lymphoma with ^{131}I anti-B1 (anti-CD20) antibody. N Eng J Med 1993; 329:459-465.
88. Divgi CR, Scott AM, Dantis L et al. Phase I radioimmunotherapy trial with I-131 CC49 in metastatic colon carcinoma. J Nuc Med 1994; (in press).
89. Kavanagh JJ. Proc 9th Int Conf Monoclonal antibody conjugates for cancer. San Diego, 1994.
90. Hird V, Maraveyas A, Snook D et al. Adjuvant therapy of ovarian cancer with radioactive monoclonal antibody. Br J Cancer 1993; 68:403-406.
91. Ward B, Mather S, Shepherd J et al. The treatment of intraperitoneal malignant disease with monoclonal antibody guided ^{131}I radiotherapy. Br J Cancer 1988: 58:658-662.
92. Jacobs AJ, Fer M, Su FM et al. A phase I trial of a rhenium 186-labeled monoclonal antibody administered intraperitoneally in ovarian carcinoma: toxicity and clinical response. Obstet Gynecol 1993; 82:586-593.
93. DeNardo GL, Lewis JP, DeNardo SJ et al. Effect of lym-1 radioimmunoconjugate on refractory chronic lymphocytic leukemia. Cancer 1994; 73:1425-1432.
94. Order SE, Sleeper AM, Stillwagon GB. Radiolabelled antibodies: results and potential in cancer therapy. Cancer Res 1990; 50 (suppl):1011s-1013s.
95. Czuczman MS, Straus DJ, Divgi CR et al. Phase I dose escalation trial of iodine 131-labeled monoclonal antibody OKB7 in patients with non-Hodgkin's lymphoma. J Clin Oncol 1993; 11:2021-2029.
96. Schwartz MA, Lovett DR, Redner A et al. Dose escalation trial of M195 labeled with iodine 131 for cytoreduction and marrow ablation in relapsed or refractory myeloid leukemias. J Clin Oncol 1993; 11:294-303.

97. Goldenberg DM, Sharkey RM, Hall TC et al. Radioimmunotherapy of B cell lymphoma with 131-I labelled LL2 (EPB-2) monoclonal antibody. Antibody Immunoconjugates Radiopharm 1991; 4:763-769.
98. Goldenberg DM. Radioimmunotherapy of thyroid carcinomas with 131-I labelled anti-CEA monoclonal antibody. Proc Int Conference on Radioimmunodetection and Radioimmunotheray, Princeton, 1994.
99. Lederman JA, Begent RHJ, Massof C et al. A phase-I study of repeated therapy with radiolabelled antibody to CEA using intermittent or continous administration of cyclosporin A to suppress the immune response. Int J Cancer 1990; (in press).
100. DeNardo SJ, Warhoe KA, O'Grady LF et al. Radioimmunotherapy with 131-I chimeric L6 in advanced breast cancer. In: Ceriani RL, ed. Breast Epithelial Antigens. New York: Plenum Press, 1991: 227-232.
101. Buchegger F. Proc 9th Int Conference of Monoclonal antibody Immunoconjugates for Cancer, San Diego, 1994.
102. Martin EW, Mojziski CM, Hinkle GH et al. Radioimmunoguided surgery: a new approach to the intraoperative detection of tumour using monoclonal antibody B72.3. Am J Surg 1988; 156:386-392.
103. Colcher D, Esteban JM, Carrasquilo JA et al. Quantitative analysis of selective radiolabelled monoclonal antibody localisation in metastatic lesions of colorectal cancer patients. Cancer Res 1987; 47:1185-1189.
104. Sears HF, Herlyn D, Steplewski Z. Effects of monoclonal antibody immunotherapy on patients with gastrointestinal adenocarcinoma. J Biol Resp Mod 1984; 3:138-150.
105. Scheinberg DA, Lovett D, Divgi CR et al. A phase I trial of monoclonal antibody M195 in acute myelogenous leukemia: specific bone marrow targeting and internalisation of radionuclide. J Clin Oncol 1991; 9:478-490.
106. Ortho multicenter transplant study group. A randomised clinical trial of OKT3 monoclonal antibody for acute rejection of cadaveric renal transpants. New Eng J Med 1985; 31:337-342.
107. Abramowicz D, Goldman M, DePauw L et al. Long term effects of prophylactic OKT3 monoclonal antibody in cadaver kidney transplantation: a single center prospective randomised study. Transplantation 1992; 54:433-437.
108. Waldmann H. Manipulation of T cell responses with monoclonal antibodies. Ann Rev Immunol 1989; 7:407-444.
109. Hale G, Waldmann H. CAMPATH-1 monoclonal antibodies in bone marrow tranplantation. J Hematotherap 1994; 3:15-31.
110. Kavanaugh AF, Davis LS, Nichols LA et al. Treatment of refractory rheumatoid arthritis with a monoclonal antibody to intercellular adhesion molecule-1. Arthritis and Rheumatism 1994; 37:992-999.

111. Soulillou JP, Cantarovich D, LeMauff B et al. Randomized control trial of a monoclonal antibody against the interleukin 2 receptor (33B3.1) as compared with rabbit anti-thymocyte globulin for prophylaxis against rejection of renal allografts. New Eng J Med 1990; 332:1175-1182.
112. Kirkman RL, Shapiro MF, Carpenter CB et al. Early experience with anti-Tac in clinical renal transplantation. Transplant Proc 1989; 21:1766-1768.
113. Friend PJ, Waldmann H, Cobbald S. The anti-IL-2 receptor monoclonal antibody YTH-906 in liver transplantation. Transplant Proc 1991; 23:1390-1392.
114. Amlot PL. Clinical use of chimeric CD7 (SDZ CHH 380) and CD25 (SDZ CHI 621) antibodies. Abstr IBC Conf Monoclonal antibodies: clinical and regulatory issues. London, 1992.
115. Maini RN, Feldmann M. Is tumour necrosis factor-α (TNFα) a potential therapeutic target in rheumatoid arthritis? Concept validation studies. Sem Clin Immunol 1993; 6:5-10.
116. Waldmann H, Cobbold S. The use of monoclonal antibodies to achieve immunological tolerance. Immunology Today 1993; 14:247-251.
117. Hering BJ, Bowatzki CC, Schultz A et al. Clinical islet transplantation-registry report accomplishments in the past and future research needs. Cell Transplant 1993; 2:269-282.
118. Brewer Y, Palmer A, Taube D et al. Effect of graft perfusion with two CD45 monoclonal antibodies on incidence of kidney allograft rejection. Lancet 1989; ii: 935-937.
119. Prentice HG, Blacklock HA, Janossy G et al. Use of anti-T cell monoclonal antibody OKT3 to prevent acute versus graft host disease in allogeneic bone marrow transplantation for acute leukemia. Lancet 1982: i:700-703.
120. Hale G, Waldmann H for CAMPATH users. Control of graft versus host disease and graft rejection by T cell depletion of donor and recipient with CAMPATH-1 antibodies. Results of matched sibling transplants for malignant diseases. Bone Marrow Transplant 1994.
121. Springer TA. Adhesion molecules of the immune system. Nature 1990; 346:425-433.
122. Ellis SG, Navetta FL, Tcheng JT et al. Safety and antiplatelet effect of murine monoclonal antibody 7E3 Fab directed against platelet glycroprotein IIb/IIIa in patients undergoing elective coronary angioplasty: an initial experience. Coron Artery Dis 1993; 4:167-175.
123. Topol EJ, Califf RM, Welsman HF et al. Randomised trial of coronary intervention with antibody against platelet IIb/IIIa integrin for the reduction of clinical restenosis: results at six months. Lancet 1994; 343:881-886.

CHAPTER 5

HUMAN MONOCLONAL ANTIBODIES

INTRODUCTION

The provision of therapeutically useful human monoclonal antibodies by hybridoma technology remains elusive due to a variety of technical limitations.[1] These can be summarized as follows:

1) Source of B cells

High affinity antibodies cannot in most cases be generated by immunization of humans. Peripheral B lymphocytes are the easiest source of cells but are difficult to use since 10% are small unstimulated cells which do not readily fuse. In addition, only a small proportion of antibody producing B cells display receptors for Epstein Barr virus (EBV) and are thus susceptible to virus induced immortalization.[2] Proliferating B cells are most susceptible both to cell fusion and EBV transformation.[3] Lymphocyte bearing organs such as spleen, tonsil and bone marrow are difficult to obtain and yield low numbers of cells.

2) Immortalization of cells

There are two classical methods for immortalizing B cells: the first is cell-cell fusion to generate human-human hybridomas or rodent-human heterohybridomas and the second is immortalization through EBV transformation.[1] Human lymphoblastoid cell lines (LCL) and heteromyelomas are now readily available as fusion partners and hybridomas secreting 10-20 μg immunoglobulin/10^6 cells can be isolated.[4] Human-human cell fusion is still a very inefficient process and rodent-human hybridomas are treacherously unstable and susceptible to chromosome loss, particularly loss of chromosomes 2, 14 and 22 which encode the light and heavy chain loci.[5-7] EBV transformed B cells have been described in innumerable publications but the vast majority are IgM secretors of low affinity and inevitably the cells are unstable and lost on subculture. The few cell lines which have survived and reached clinical trials have been derived from optimally immunized donors as will be discussed later.

3) Large scale production

Yields of antibody in the range of 10-20 μg per 10^6 cells are insufficient for the cost effective manufacture of a human therapeutic. These yields contrast strongly with production levels from murine hybridomas or genetically engineered humanized antibodies where yields are 10-fold higher. Furthermore, EBV transformed human-mouse heterohybridomas or human-human hybridomas cannot be grown in large scale culture to the very high cell concentrations achievable with murine hybridoma NS0 cells, CHO cells or rat YB20 cells which are used for provision of genetically engineered antibodies. It is doubtful then whether many of the human monoclonals currently in advanced clinical trials will be capable of meeting market requirements without further development of genetically recombinant versions. Such work is likely to delay their appearance on the market by several years.

Human monoclonals from mouse-human heterohybridomas have the additional problem that these cell lines secrete a mixture of antibody species including murine heavy (H) chains/human light (L) chains, human H/murine L and murine H/murine L derived from the cell fusion partner. Sophisticated purification procedures are required to separate intact human antibody species.

Recombinant DNA technology and bacteriophage display libraries offer alternative routes to human monoclonals but the breadth of application of these technologies to provide therapeutics remains to be proven (chapter 9).

Alternative cell biological approaches remain worthy of pursuit and important improvements and novel methodologies have been developed in recent years. It is these advances which are reviewed in this chapter.

ISOLATION OF HIGH AFFINITY HUMAN B CELLS

Selection of Donors

The vast majority of high affinity monoclonal antibodies have been derived from donors who were either vaccinated or had been naturally exposed to immunogen. It is not surprising then that 4/6 of those monoclonal antibodies in clinical trial are predominantly anti-infectives (Table 5.1).

Many attempts have been made to identify tumor reactive human monoclonal antibodies from patients. The literature suggests that peripheral blood lymphocytes (PBLs) are the least efficient source since B cells from patients with cancer are generally not tumor immune with many being suppresser cells.[8] Lymph nodes appear to be the best source but the majority of identified B cells react with common cytoplasmic or cytoskeletal human components.[9] Regional lymph nodes draining tumors are generally enlarged and B lymphocytes can develop germinal centers of antibody secreting B cells. These are proving a more productive source of tumor reactive antibodies.[10,11] One example is the isolation of the hybridoma cell line designated Monopharm-C, an IgM with immunoreactivity restricted to malignancies of epithelial origin.[12] Recent years has seen progress in active specific immunotherapy (ASI) whereby patients are immunized with autologous tumor and Bacillus Calmette and Guerin (BCG) vaccine.[13] Human IgM monoclonals specific for colorectal tumors have been isolated from patients immunized in this way.[14]

Table 5.1. Human monoclonal antibodies in clinical trials

Antibody	Antigen	Status of trial	Reference
HA-1A	LPS	Phase III	45
MSL-109	CMV(gH)	Phase II	46-48
89-104	CMV(gB)	Phase I	48
C23	CMV(gB)	Phase I/II	61
OST 577	Hepatitis B	Phase I/II	49
16.88	Colorectal cancer	Phase I/II	58
	Breast cancer	Phase I/II	60
	Metasatic melanoma GD2	Phase I/II	59

In Vitro Immunization

To overcome the severe limitations imposed upon in vivo immunization, several methods for effective in vitro immunization of human B cells have been described[3] and give rise to populations of human B cells enriched for secretion of antibodies against the target antigen. Human peripheral blood lymphocytes are the cells of choice and the breadth of antigen specific cells which have been identified is summarized in Table 5.2. The antigenicity of small molecules has been enhanced by conjugation to carriers such as keyhole limpet hemocyanin,[15] tetanus toxoid[16] and silica beads.[17] In one example, the cancer associated antigen bombesin was conjugated to sepharose beads and used to select B cells which bound to tumor cells.[16] B cells recognizing macromolecular antigens have also been isolated by addition of whole target cells to in vitro immunization systems.[18] More effective immunization can be achieved in some cases by the addition of cytokines or growth factors such as IL-1, IL-2 and B cell growth factor (BCGF).[3] It is thought that they act by activating B cells to enter a phase of growth cycle more susceptible to antigen stimulation.

An important advance was the recognition of the need to deplete T suppressor cells from cultures[19] and provide polyclonal cell stimulants such as pokeweed mitogen and IL-2.[20] A combination of these factors has now permitted the primary antigenic stimulation of human splenocytes to generate IgM secreting cells and stimulate secondary response to yield IgG secretors.[21]

Table 5.2. Antigens which have been used for the in vitro immunization of B cells

Antigen	
Human mammary carcinomas	Prostatic acid phosphatase
Human prostate	Rhesus D
Lung cancer antigens	Tetanus toxid
Melanoma cells	Influenza
Cellular antigens	Tetanus toxoid
Bombesin	Hepatitis B surface antigen
Cytomegalovirus	Herpes simplex virus I and II
Varicella zoster	Human immunodeficiency virus
J5 endotoxin	*Neisseria meningitidis*

Adapted from: Glassy MC. Production methods for generating human monoclonal antibodies. Hum Antibody Hybridomas 1993; 4:154-165; Koda K, Glassy MC. In vitro immunisation for the production of human monoclonal antibody. Hum Antibody Hybridomas 1990; 1:15-22; and Borrebaeck C. Human Mabs produced by primary in vitro immunization. Immunology Today 1988; 9:355-359.

Antigen specific B cell cultures provided by these methods do not normally survive in culture for extended periods of time but extensive studies with a plethora of cytokines and growth factors is slowly defining culture conditions for long term cell survival. In particular, IL-4 and CD40 stimulation permit survival in culture for up to one year.[22]

Despite these improvements, the human monoclonals so developed are normally low-to-intermediate affinity IgM antibodies and are not directly suitable as therapeutics.[19] It has been argued that such cultures can be used as the starting material for affinity maturation through in vitro mutagenesis[23] though the possibility of generating immunogenic epitopes on the antibody must be considered.

Immunization of Transplanted SCID Mice

Mice with severe combined immunodeficiency disease (SCID) lack functional T and B cells due to a mutation affecting the immunoglobulin recombinase gene.[24-26] These mice accept a wide range of human tissue grafts including fetal liver, bone marrow, thymus and mature human peripheral blood lymphocytes which survive for up to two years and continue to secrete human IgM and IgG.[27-29]

SCID mice have been successfully populated with human PBLs (hu-PBL-SCID) from unimmunized, immunized and diseased patients. In the latter case, the transfer of lymphocytes from patients with primary biliary cirrhosis,[30] rheumatoid arthritis and SLE[31,32] have been described with, in some cases, the transfer of some of the pathological symptoms. Transferred PBLs have been successfully infected in vivo with EBV[33,34] and HIV.[35]

This system has now been developed for active immunization. The immunization with tetanus toxoid of SCID mice which have been populated with human PBLs resulted in the specific elevation of the level of human anti-tetanus antibody[36] demonstrating antigen-specific stimulation of human B cell proliferation in vivo. More recently, the stimulation of a secondary response has been described.[37] In this study, PBLs derived from an unimmunized donor were transferred into SCID mice which were then immunized with hepatitis B core (Hbc) antigen. A small proportion of the mice showed a strong IgG anti-Hbc response with serum antibody levels 10^2 to 10^3 fold higher than the donor. This work also demonstrated that one can populate a SCID mouse with PBLs from an individual who had been exposed to antigen in the distant past but who is no longer producing antibody and, by immunization of the SCID, one can recover the memory B cell population. This may offer a method of identifying disease related B cells in a patient's history.

Immortalization of B Cells

Traditional methods of EBV transformation and hybrid cell fusion are still the main techniques for the immortalization of B cells. In recent years there has been increased variety in choice of fusion partners.[4] The technology has also been extended by the use of electroporation[38] to introduce gene vectors carrying immortalizing oncogenes directly into human B cells[39] or through the use of electrofusion to generate human-human hybridomas.[40] Such methods continue to provide monoclonal cell lines (Table 5.3) but relatively few have had the required cell stability and acceptable antibody yield to be carried through to clinical studies.

Rescue of Antibody Genes from Single B Cells

A promising methodology to overcome the instability of immortalized B cells is the early rescue of the monoclonal heavy and light chain genes from a small clonal B cell population or from single B cells.[41] The method is analogous to that described in chapter 7 for the construction of immunoglobulin libraries except that PCR based amplification of the heavy and light chains is carried out within a single permeabilized cell in such a way that the heavy and light genes become covalently linked to ensure retention of the B cell heavy and light chain association (Fig. 5.1). The method is, however, technically demanding and requires further development.

CLINICAL STUDIES WITH HUMAN MONOCLONAL ANTIBODIES

Those human monoclonal antibodies which have entered clinical trials are summarized in Table 5.1. The low number compared to Table 5.3 emphasizes the technical difficulties involved.

Anti-Infectives

HA-1A

HA-1A was raised by immunization of a volunteer with *E. coli* J-5 vaccine and immortalization of B cells by EBV transformation followed by heterohybridoma generation though fusion of the hu-

Table 5.3. Antigens recognized by human monoclonal antibodies

Viruses		
Cytomegalovirus	Influenza	HIV-1
Epstein-Barr virus	Rabies	Rubella
Hepatitis A,B,C	Varicella zoster	Measles
Human T cell leukemia virus	Herpes simplex I, II	
Bacteria		
Haemophilus influenzae	Gram-negative endotoxin	Diphteria toxin
Tetanus toxid	Mycobacterium	Cholera toxin
Niesseria meningitidis	*Pneumococcus leprae*	Chlamydia
Pseudomonas aeruginosa	*P. aeruginosa* exotoxin A	
Blood cell antigens		
Rhesus c,C,D,e,E,G,J	Blood groups A	
HLA-B and DQ	Forsmann antigen	
Tumor antigens		
Bladder carcinoma	Brain glioma	Breast carcinoma
Cervical carcinoma	Colorectal carcinoma	Gastric carcinoma
Chronic lymphocytic leukemia	Lung carcinoma	Lymphoma
Myeloma	Myeloid leukemia	Renal carcinoma
Prostatic carcinoma	Stomach carcinoma	
Autoantigens		
Astrocytes	Cytoskeletal proteins	ss and ds DNA
Endothelial cells	Myelin basic sheath	Golgi apparatus
Nuclear and nucleolar antigens	Nerve axons	Neurons
Pancreatic cells	Parathyroid	Pituitory
Platelets	Prostatic acid phosphatase	Sperm
Sperm coating protein	Stratified squamous epithelium	
Thyroglobulin	Thyroid follicle	Vimetin
Rheumatoid factor	Bombesin	

Adapted from: Glassy MC. Production methods for generating human monoclonal antibodies. Hum Antibody Hybridomas 1993; 4:154-165; Boyd JE, James K. Human monoclonal antibodies: their potential, problems and prospects. Adv Biotech Processes 1989; 11:1-43; andLarrick JW. Potential of monoclonal antibodies as pharmacological agents. Pharmacol Rev 1989; 41:539-557.

man lymphoblastoid cell line with a murine hybridoma.[44] Though described as a human monoclonal, the antibody consists of human VH and VL domains but the J chain is of murine origin. This IgM antibody has undergone aggressive clinical development by Centocor Inc. and is intended for therapy against sepsis. The clinical progress of this antibody has provided a salutary lesson that care and attention to detail during clinical studies, cautious interpretation of data and the need for thorough study of the mode

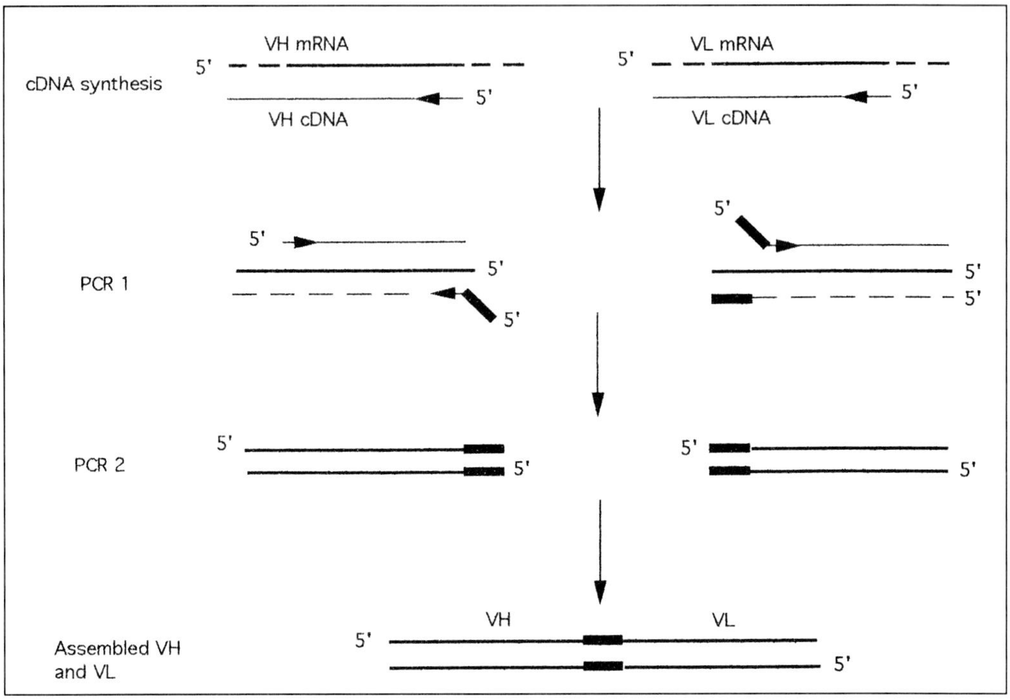

Fig. 5.1. In-cell PCR amplification of VH and Vκ. Oligonucleotide primers for the preferential conversion of VH and Vκ mRNA into cDNA are infused into permeabilized hybridoma cells and then additional primers introduced to effect PCR amplification. The 5' primers of VH and Vκ carry a complementary nucleotide sequence so that during the PCR reactions a single chain Fv genetic construct will be assembled. This ensures that the original VH/Vκ combination is retained. Adapted from: Embleton MJ, Gorochov G, Jones PT et al. In-cell PCR from mRNA: amplifying and linking the rearranged immunogloubulin heavy and light chain V genes within single cells. Nucleic Acid Res 1992; 20:3831-3837.

of action of a therapeutic are pre-requisites for success. HA-1A has a broad specificity for naturally occurring rough mutants of gram negative bacteria, its specificity being directed to the lipid A domain of lipopolysaccharide. Despite being an IgM, it shows high binding affinity of the order of 10^{-8} M for bacteria previously treated with antibiotics to expose the antigen. The mechanism of action is not clearly understood but it was surmised that the antibody, by binding either to the bacterial cell surface or to the circulating LPS endotoxin fragments, activated complement. The C3b fragment generated was then proposed to form a tertiary complex with HA-1A/LPS which bound to the CR1 receptors on red blood cells. This cellular binding could prevent LPS from reacting with effector cells such as macrophages, thus blocking initiation of the cytokine cycle which results in septic shock.[44]

The safety of HA-1A was evaluated in five phase I trials ranging from single to five doses of 100 mg.[45] In over 4,000 patients the most common side effect was hypotension during infusion. No anti-HA-1A antibody response was identified. In the initial phase II trial the data was interpreted to demonstrate a reduction in mortality from 47% (with placebo) to 30% in 200 cases with documented gram negative bacteremia. HA-1A was then made available on a compassionate-use basis in the United States whereby a physician could contact Centocor for a course of HA-1A. Four thousand patients were enrolled on this basis. To interpret the data, since there was not a concurrent placebo group, the expected mortality was calculated from historical data. Interpretation was complex since the baseline factors which defined the disease state were different between the historical and treated groups. The data was again interpreted as demonstrating a reduction in mortality due to HA-1A. A more focused phasc III trial is currently ongoing in patients with meningococcemia.

CYTOMEGALOVIRUS

MSL 109

MSL 109 (originally developed and trialed by Sandoz, but now licensed to Protein Design Laboratories) is a human IgG_1/κ monoclonal antibody specific for the glycoprotein gH which is a major neutralizing determinant of human cytomegalovirus (CMV). The antibody neutralizes all tested strains of CMV with an ED50 in the range of 1.25 μg/ml. Anti-gH antibodies in general prevent viral entry into cells. In toxicology studies in adult and neonatal primates, up to 16 mg/kg dose levels have been administered and no clinical or pathological abnormalities detected. Two clinical trials have been completed in patients undergoing allogeneic or autologous bone marrow transplantation. In one study,[46] eight patients received doses of 0.5 and 2 mg/kg every two weeks for 12 weeks. No toxic symptoms or human anti-human antibody (HAHA) response were noted though the patients were immunosuppressed. The serum half life of six days was much lower than normal for human antibodies but this is likely to be attributable to the increased protein catabolism which occurs after such transplantation. In a second study,[47] 15 patients received 0.05, 0.25 or 0.5 mg/kg every three weeks for six months with minimal side effects reported and no HAHA response. A serum half life of up to 16.5 days was reported. Efficacy was not reported in these phase I studies. Two phase I/II clinical trials in AIDS patients have been reported.[48] Patients received up to 2 mg/kg MSL 109 every two weeks for 24 weeks with comparative controls receiving 3 mg/kg doses of IVIG. Only one mild headache was reported as an adverse effect in one patient and none of the patients developed a HAHA response. The serum half lives were of the order of two weeks. Efficacy analysis has not been completely reported. In the second study, MSL 109 was given concurrently with ganciclovir or foscarnet to AIDS patients with documented CMV retinitis. The median time to progression of retinitis was 200 days in patients given MSL 109 compared with 100 days calculated from historical controls. Further trials are planned, though a major limiting factor is likely to be the supply of material from the low level of production by the cell line.

89-104

This antibody, also developed by Sandoz, neutralizes CMV infection through interaction with glycoprotein gB of CMV.[46] Five patients undergoing bone marrow transplantation received this antibody with no deleterious effects.[48] In view of the advanced development of MSL 109, this antibody is unlikely to be tested further in the near future. Also, strain variation within the gB protein of CMV is significant, raising the possibility that anti-gB monoclonal antibodies would not neutralize all clinical isolates.

Hepatitis B

OST 577

OST 577 is an antibody with specificity for hepatitis B surface (S) antigen which has been trialed in post-liver transplant patients by Sandoz though the antibody has now been licensed to Protein Design Laboratories. Five patients received up to 40 doses of between 0.15 and 0.5 mg/kg for up to 92 weeks.[49] The serum half life was of the order of 20 days and no HAHA response was noted. Re-infection of the patients was prevented for over one year.

HIV

Initial studies with antibody based therapy have been with polyclonal sera from healthy HIV infected individuals. Small open label, uncontrolled studies were carried out in advanced AIDS patients with inconclusive results.[50-52] However, data from well controlled Phase II studies have shown polyclonal sera to be active in AIDS treatment.[53] In one study, 86 patients showed a significant reduction in low $CD4^+$ cell counts and AIDS defining clinical events. While the control group had a mean of 1.25 AIDS defining events per patient, the treatment group had 0.43 events per patient. There were seven deaths in the treated group and 11 in the control group. It was concluded that while antiserum did not result in clinical improvement, it did slow progression of disease.

A number of heterohybridoma cell lines producing human antibodies against the V3 loop and CD4 binding domain of HIV have been described.[54] Anti-V3 loop monoclonal antibodies show greater virus neutralization activity in vitro and are the most promising candidates for clinical trial.

ANTI-RHESUS D

The use of anti-rhesus D (Rh D) monoclonal antibodies to replace polyclonal antiserum for immune prophylaxis of haemolytic disease of the newborn due to Rh D-incompatible pregnancies would seem to represent an early opportunity for monoclonal antibody based therapy, particularly since human anti-Rh D monoclonal antibodies are relatively easy to derive and have been available for over 10 years.[55] However, the Rh D antigen is still poorly understood and many anti-Rh D monoclonals have cross reactivity with normal tissue.[56] Two anti-Rh D monoclonal antibodies have been shown to cause accelerated clearance of coated red blood cells in Rhesus positive male volunteers.[57] Phase II clinical trials are likely to be delayed due to the sensitivity of testing a new product on the newborn.

ANTI-CANCER MONOCLONAL ANTIBODIES

IgM monoclonals against cytoplasmic (28A32; 16.88) and cell surface (28A32) components of colon carcinoma cells have been obtained from colon cancer patients vaccinated with autologous tumor and BCG.[14] In a phase I study, patients with metastatic colorectal carcinomas were given a single intravenous injection of ^{131}I labeled antibody (5 mCi/8 μg). Tumor uptake was observed in 12/16 patients given 28A32 and 9/12 given 16.88. The average retention time in tumor nodules was 17 days with the smallest tumors detectable being 2 cm in diameter. Tumor to normal tissue uptake ratios of about 10 to 1 were noted with 16.88.[58] None of the patients given 16.88 developed an antibody response but a low titer of anti-28A32 developed in 4/16 patients given this antibody. This low antibody response did not seem to affect serum half life. 28A32 was derived from a human-mouse heterohybri-doma while 16.88 was an EBV transformed cell line and this may account for the different immunogenicity profiles. Additional studies with 16.88, including a single dose of up to 1 g of antibody in colorectal patients, showed tumor uptake in 80% of patients but no tumor regressions were reported.[59] Regression of cutaneous metastatic melanomas have been observed after intralesional injection of a human monoclonal to ganglioside GD2.[60] Ten breast cancer patients have been treated with three different IgM monoclonals at single doses up to 22 mg but no tumor regression was noted.[61]

References

1. James K, Bell GT. Human monoclonal antibody production. Current status and future prospects. J Immunol Methods 1987; 100:5-40.
2. Crain MJ, Sanders SK, Butler JL et al. Epstein-Barr virus preferentially induces proliferation of primed B-cells.. J Immunol 1989; 143:1543-1548.
3. Glassy MC. Production methods for generating human monoclonal antibodies. Hum Antibody Hybridomas 1993; 4:154-165.
4. Boyd JE, James K. Human monoclonal antibodies: their potential, problems and prospects. Adv Biotech Processes 1989; 11:1-43.
5. Schlom J, Wunderlich D, Teramoto YA. Generation of human monoclonal antibodies reactive with human mammary carcinoma cells. Proc Nat Acad Sci 1980; 77:6841-6845.
6. Lowe DH, Handley H, Schmidt J. A human monoclonal antibody reactive with human prostate. J Urol 1984; 132:780-785.
7. Sikora K, Wright R. Human monoclonal antibodies to lung cancer antigens. Br J Cancer 1981; 43:696-702.
8. Glassy MC, Dillman RO. Molecular biotherapy with human monoclonal antibodies. Mol Biother 1988; 1:7-13.
9. Cote RJ, Morrissey DM, Houghton AN et al. Specificity analysis of human monoclonal antibodies reactive with cell surface and intracellular antigens. Proc Nat Acad Sci 1986; 83:2959-2963.
10. Sikora K, Alderson T, Nethersall A et al. Tumour localisation by human monoclonal antibodies. Med Oncol & Tumour Pharmacother 1985; 2:77-86.
11. Banerjee D, Karim R, Hearn SA et al. Human monoclonal antibodies to neuroendocrine granules derived from tumour-infiltrating lymphocytes isolated from a primitive neuroectodermal tumour. Hum Antibody Hybridomas 1990; 1:55-63.

12. Koda K, Glassy MC, Chang HR. Generation of human monoclonal antibodies against colon cancer. Arch Surg 1990; 125: 1591-1597.
13. Hoover HC, Surdyke MG, Dangel RB et al. Prospectively randomised trial of adjuvant active specific immunotherapy for human colorectal cancer. Cancer 1985; 55:1236-1243.
14. Haspel MV, McCabe RP, Pomato N et al. Generation of tumour cell-reactive human monoclonal antibodies using periphral blood lymphocytes from actively immunised colorectal carcinoma patients. Cancer Res 1986; 45:3951-3961.
15. Wasserman RL, Budens RD, Thaxton ES. *In vitro* stimulation prior to fusion generates antigen binding human-human hybridomas. J Immunol Methods 1986; 93:275-283.
16. Ho M-K, Rand N, Murray J et al. *In vitro* immunisation of human lymphocytes. 1. Production of human monoclonal antibodies against bombesin and tetanus toxoid. J Immunol 1985; 135: 3831-3838.
17. Olsson L, Brams P. Human-human hybridoma technology. Five years of technical improvements and its application in cancer biology. In: Engleman EG, Foung SKH, Larrick J et al. eds. Human Hybridomas and Monoclonal Antibodies. New York: Plenum, 1985;227-244.
18. Hulette CM, Effros RB, Waford RL. Immunisation of normal human splenocytes *in vitro* to produce human monoclonal antibodies to cellular antigens. Tissue Antigens 1987; 30:25-33.
19. Borrebaeck CAK. *In vitro* Immunisation in Hybridoma Technology. New York: Elsevier, 1988.
20. Koda K, Glassy MC. *In vitro* immunisation for the production of human monoclonal antibody. Hum Antibody Hybridomas 1990; 1:15-22.
21. Boerner P, Lafond R, Lu W-Z et al. Production of antigen-specific human monoclonal antibodies from *in vitro* primed human splenocytes. J Immunol 1991; 147:86-95.
22. Banchereau J, de Paoli P, Valle A et al. Long term human B cell lines dependent on interleukin-4 and antibody to CD40. Science 1991; 251:70-72.
23. Glasser SM, Yelton DE, Huse WD et al. Antibody engineering by codon-based mutagenesis in a filamentous phage vector system. J Immunol 1992; 149:3903-3913.
24. Bosma GC, Custer RP, Bosma MJ. A severe combined immunodeficiency mutation in the mouse. Nature 1983; 301:527-530.
25. Schuler WI, Weiler J, Schuler A et al. Rearrangement of antigen receptor genes is defective in mice with severe combined immunodeficiency. Cell 1986; 46:963-972.
26. Fulop GM, Phillips RA. The Scid mutation in mice causes a general defect in DNA repair. Nature 1990; 347:479-482.

27. Phillis RA, Jewett MAS, Gallie BL. Growth of human tumours in immunodeficient scid mice and nude mice. The Scid mouse: characterisation and potential uses. Curr Topics Microbiol Immunol 1989; 152: 259-263.
28. Mosier DE, Gulizia RJ, Baird SM et al. Transfer of a functional immune system to mice with severe combined immunodeficiency . Nature 1988; 335:256-259.
29. Duchosal MA, Eming SA, McConahey PJ et al. Long term human serologic evolution associated with the xenogeneic transfer of human peripheral blood leukocytes into SCID mice. Celular Immunology 1992; 139:468-477.
30. Krams SM, Dorshkind K, Gershwin ME. Generation of biliary lesions after transfer of human lymphocytes into Scid mice. J Exp Med 1989; 170:1919-1930.
31. Tighe H, Silveman GJ, Kozin F et al. Autoantibody production by severe combined immunodeficient mice reconstituted with synovial cells from rheumatoid arthritis patients. Eur J Immunol 1990; 20:1843-1848.
32. Duchosal MA, McConahey PJ, Robinson CA et al. Transfer of human systemic lupus erythromatosus in Scid mice. J Exp Med 1990; 172:985-988.
33. Cannon MJ, Pisa P, Fox RI et al. Epstein-Barr virus induces aggressive lymphoproliferative disorders of human B cell origin in Scid/hu chimeric mouse. J Clin Invest 1990; 85:1333-1337.
34. Okano M, Taguchi Y, Naamine H et al. Characterisation of Epstein-Barr virus induced lymphoproliferation derived from human peripheral blood mononuclear cells transferred to severe combined immunodeficient mice. Am J Pathol 1990; 137:517-522.
35. Mosier DE, Gulizia RJ, Baird SM et al. Human immmunodeficiency virus infection of human PBL-SCID mice. Science 1991; 251:791-794.
36. Carlson R, Martensson C, Kalliomaki S et al. Human peripheral blood lymphocytes transplanted into Scid mice constitute an *in vivo* culture system exhibiting several parameters found in a normal human immune response and are a source of immunocytes for the production of human monoclonal antibodies. J Immunol 1992; 148:1065-1071.
37. Duchosal MA, Eming SA, Fischer P et al. Immunisation of Hu-PBL-SCID mice and the rescue of human monoclonal Fab fragments through combinatorial libraries. Nature 1992; 355:258-262.
38. Chang DC, Chassy BM, Saunders JA et al. eds. Handbook of Electroporation and Electrofusion. Orlando: Academic Press, 1991.
39. Mally MI, Glassy MC. Generating immortalised Ig-secreting human lymphocytes by recombinant DNA technology. In: Borrebaeck CAK, Hagen I, eds. Electromanipulation in Hybridoma Technology. New York: Stockton Press, 1990:71-88.

40. Steenbakkers PG, Van Meel FCM, Olijve W. A new approach to the generation of human x murine antibody producing hybridomas. J Immunol Method. 1992; 152:69-77.
41. Embleton MJ, Gorochov G, Jones PT et al. In-cell PCR from mRNA: amplifying and linking the rearranged immunogloubulin heavy and light chain V genes within single cells. Nucleic Acid Res 1992; 20:3831-3837.
42. Larrick JW. Potential of monoclonal antibodies as pharmacological agents. Pharmacol Rev 1989; 41:539-557.
43. Borrebaeck C. Human Mabs produced by primary *in vitro* immunization. Immunology Today 1988; 9:355-359.
44. Baumgarther JD. Monoclonal anti-endotoxin antibodies for the treatment of gram negative bacteremia and septic shock. Eur J Clin Microbiol Inf Dis 1990; 9:711-716.
45. Smith C, Wortel C, Dixon W et al. Monoclonal antibody HA-1A for gram negative shock. Lancet 1991; 338:695-696.
46. Aulitsky WE, Schult TF, Tilg H et.al. Human monoclonal antibodies neutralising cytomegalovirus (CMV) for the prophylaxis of CMV disease: report of a phase I trial in bone marrow transplant recipients. J Infect Dis 1991; 163:1344-1347.
47. Drobyski WR, Gottlieb M, Carrigan D et al. Phase I study of safety and pharmacokinetics of a human antimegalovirus monoclonal antibody in allogeneic bone marrow transplant recipients. Transplantation 1991. 51;1190-1196
48. Nadler PI, Wood DL, Ostberg L et al. The use of human and genetically engineered humanised antibodies for the prophylaxis and treatment of cytomegalovirus infection. Transplant Immunol Letter 1994; IX:6-9.
49. Cornett JB. Clinical results with humanised and human monoclonals. In: Kobayashi T, Kitagawa Y, Ougamura K et al. eds. Animal Cell Technology. Dordrecht: Academic Pub. 1993; 6:63-73.
50. Jackson GG, Perkins JT, Rubenis M et al. Passive immunoneutralising of human immunodeficiency virus in patients with advanced AIDS. Lancet 1988: ii:647-652.
51. Karpas A, Hill F, Youle M et al. Effects of passive immunisation in patients with the acquired immunodeficiency syndrome-related complex and acquired immunodeficiency syndrome. Proc Nat Acad Sci 1988; 85:9234-9237.
52. Osther K et al. PASSHIV-I treatment of patients with HIV-I infection. A preliminary report of a phase I trial of hyperimmune porcine immunoglobulin to HIV-1 AIDS 1992; 6:1457-1464.
53. Jacobson JM, Colman N, Ostrow NA et al. Passive immunotherapy in treatment of advanced HIV infection. J Infec Dis 1993; 168:298-305. Erratum; J Infec Dis 1993; 168:298-305.
54. Gorny M, Conley AJ, Karwowski S et al. Neutralisation of diverse human immunodeficiency virus type I variants by an anti-V3 human monoclonal antibody. J Virol 1992; 66:7538-7542.

55. Crawford DH, Barlow MJ, Harrison JF et al. Production of human monoclonal antibody to Rhesus D antigen. Lancet 1983; i:386-388.
56. Thompson KM, Sutherland J, Barden G et al. Human monoclonal antibodies specific for blood group antigens demonstrate multispecific properties characteristic of natural autoantibodies. Immunology 1992; 76:146-157.
57. Thomson A, Contreras M, Gorick B et al. Clearance of RhD-positive red cells with monoclonal anti-D. Lancet 1990; 336:1147-1150.
58. Haisma HJ, Pinedo HM, Kessel MAP. Human IgM monoclonal antibody 16.88: pharmacokinetics and immunogenicity in colorectal cancer patients. J Nat Cancer Inst 1991; 83:1813-1819.
59. Irie RF, Morton DL. Regression of cutaneous metastatic melanoma by intralesional injection with human monoclonal antibody to ganglioside GD2. Proc Nat Acad Sci 1986; 83:8694-869.
60. Ryan KP, Dillman, RO, DeNardo SL et al. Breast cancer imaging with In-111 human IgM monclonal antibodies. Radiology 1988: 167:71-75.
61. Mashudo Y. Passive immunoprophylaxis with human monoclonal antibodies. In: Ellis RW ed. Vaccines: New Approaches to Immunoglobulin Problems. Boston: Butterworth 1992:405-430.

CHAPTER 6

HUMANIZED ANTIBODIES

INTRODUCTION

As discussed in chapter 4, the therapeutic use of mouse monoclonal antibodies is limited by (a) short serum half life (b) poor utilization of the constant region of murine antibody by human effector functions and (c) human anti-mouse antibody response (HAMA). Conversion of the mouse monoclonal antibody to a mouse-human chimeric antibody (chapter 4) provided a solution to (b) and a partial solution to (a) and (c).

The major advance, however, has been the ability to humanize rodent antibodies, a methodology which provides a monoclonal antibody which retains the antigen binding specificity of the rodent but is encoded by 95% human genetic information. Over 80 rodent antibodies have been humanized since the first description of the technique in 1986[1] and at least eight have entered clinical trial.[2,3] This chapter summarizes the methodology's scope and the progress which has been made in developing this important group of therapeutic antibodies. A number of reviews have been published in the last few years.[4-8]

STRUCTURE OF HUMANIZED ANTIBODIES

The aim of antibody humanization is the transfer of the antigen binding domains from a rodent antibody into a human framework. It can be seen from Figure 6.1 that CDRs extend outwards from the relatively conserved framework scaffold of the rest of the molecule, giving the opportunity to mount murine CDRs upon a human scaffold and possibly retain antigen binding affinity. A basic

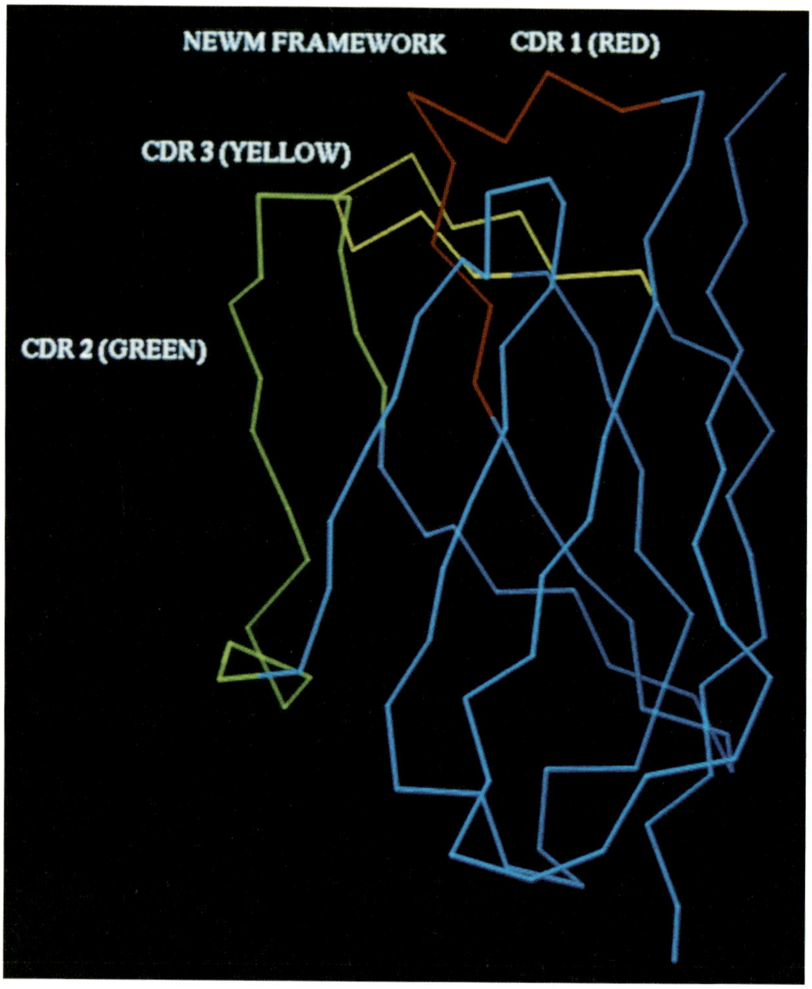

Fig. 6.1. Computer graphic model of VH of antibody NEWM showing CDR1 (red), CDR2 (green) CDR3 (yellow), as loops extending outwards from the framework backbone (blue).

outline of the methodology of 'CDR grafting' is presented in Figure 6.2 whereby the nucleotide sequences representing the six CDRs, as defined by Kabat,[9] are substituted for the corresponding CDRs in a cloned human antibody gene (see below). However, the transferred CDRs must assume their correct conformation to bind antigen and this depends upon key CDR-framework residue interactions. Thus, certain murine framework residues must also be introduced into the human framework to restore antigen binding affinity. This latter step will be referred to as reshaping the human antibody.

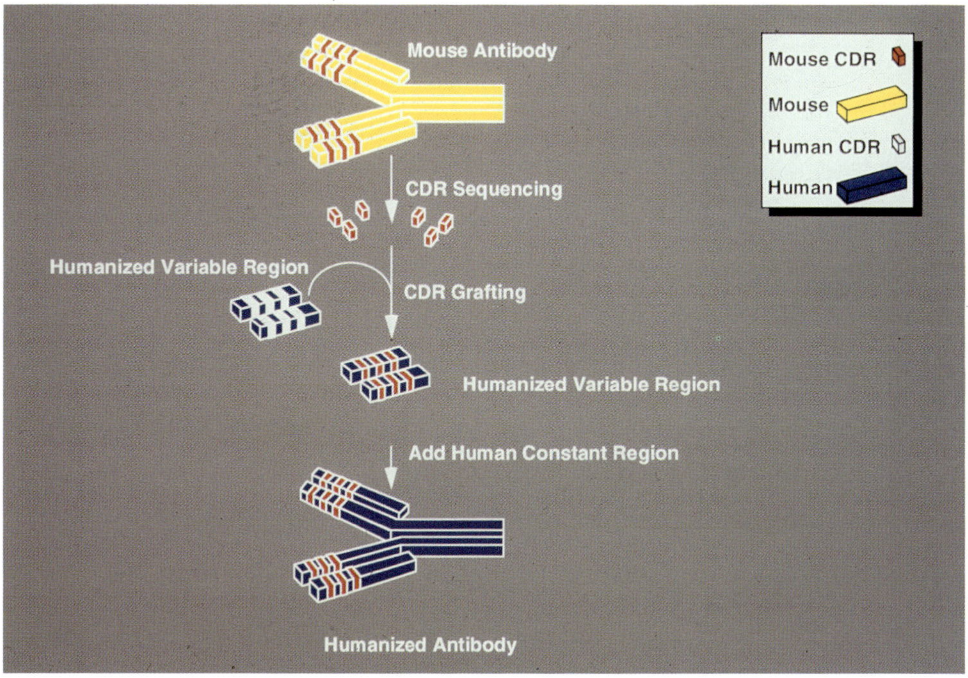

Fig. 6.2. Schematic diagram outlining the humanization of a rodent antibody in which the CDRs of a human antibody are replaced by those of a rodent antibody with the desired specificity.

CDR GRAFTING

The steps involved, starting with a murine hybridoma cell line have been described in detail[10,11] and can be summarized as follows (Fig. 6.3):

1) Cloning immunoglobulin variable region segments

mRNA from a hybridoma cell line is transcribed into cDNA. Since there is a high degree of conservation of nucleotide sequence at the 5' ends of both VH and Vκ genes and the CH1/CL genes 3' to the J regions, synthetic oligonucleotide primers can be designed to selectively amplify the VH and VL genes using the polymerase chain reaction (PCR).[12] These PCR products are purified and cloned for nucleotide sequencing.

2) Delineation of CDRs

Deduced nucleotide sequences are translated into their corresponding amino acid sequences and compared with consensus sequences of murine Ig VH and VL both to identify the murine family of origin and define the CDRs or hypervariable loops.[9] An example is shown in Table 6.1.

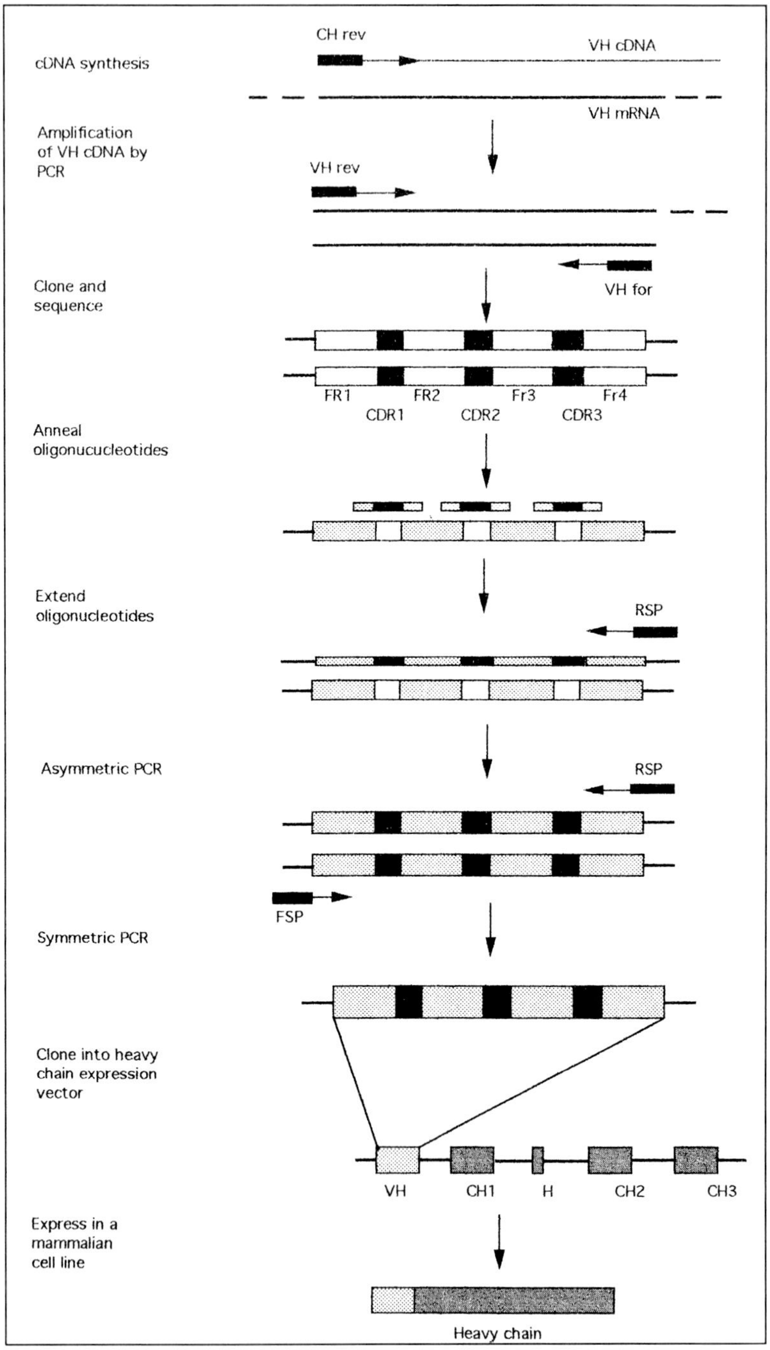

Fig. 6.3. Method of CDR grafting a VH domain gene. mRNA is isolated from a rodent hybridoma cell line and first strand cDNA synthesized by priming using a CH1 domain gene segment specific primer. This cDNA is then amplified using primers which anneal at either end of the variable domain gene. The PCR product is cloned and sequenced and this information used to generate three oligonucleotides based on the reverse complementary sequence of the monoclonal antibody VH CDR sequences as defined by Kabat and colleagues.[9] In addition, each primer has 5' and 3' 12 base flanking sequences which are designed to allow the primer to anneal to the human VH domain gene of choice. The human VH domain gene is present in a single stranded closed circular cloning vector such as M13. The oligonucleotide primers are annealed, extended and ligated to form a complete circular strand. At this stage one strand of DNA contains the original human CDRs while the complementary strand contains the rodent CDR sequences. Asymmetric PCR is carried out using the universal reverse sequencing primer (RSP) to preferentially amplify the mutant strand. This strand is further amplified by symmetric PCR using the universal forward (FSP) and reverse primers. After sequencing to verify the presence of all three rodent CDRs in the human framework the humanized VH domain is cloned into an expression vector and co-expressed with a similarly humanized light chain V domain in a mammalian cell line.

Table 6.1. Alignment of (a) the VH and (b) Vκ amino acid sequences for a monoclonal antibody (3α4D10)

(a)

```
                   10        20        30        40
                    |         |         |         |
3α4D10VH  QVQLQESGAELVRSGASVRLSCTASGFNIKDYYIHWVKQRPDQG
          :VQLQ:SGAELV::GASV:LSCTASGFNIKD Y:HWVKQRP:QG
MUVHIIC   EVQLQQSGAELVKPGASVKLSCTASGFNIKDTYMHWVKQRPEQG

                50        60        70        80
                 |         |         |         |
3α4D10VH  LEWIGWIDPENVDTEYAPKFQGKATMTADTSSNTAYLQLSSLTS
          LEWIG:IDP.N :T.Y.PKFQGKAT:TADTSSNTAYLQLSSLTS
MUVHIIC   LEWIGRIDPANGNTKYDPKFQGKATITADTSSNTAYLQLSSLTS

            90        100        110
             |         |          |
3α4D10VH  VDTAVYYCNALDYSDYPFDYWGQGTTVTVSS
           DTAVYYC.   Y. Y:.DYWGQGT:VTVSS
MUVHIIC   EDTAVYYCARGYYDYYAMDYWGQGTSVTVSS
```

(b)

```
                   10        20        30        40
                    |         |         |         |
3α4D10Vκ  DIQLTQSPASLAVSLGQRATISCRTSKSVSTSGYSYMHWYQQKPG
          DI LTQSPASLAVSLGQRATISCR:S.SV.. G S:MHWYQQKPG
MUVκIII   DIVLTQSPASLAVSLGQRATISCRASESVDXYGNSFMHWYQQKPG

                50        60        70        80        90
                 |         |         |         |         |
3α4D10Vκ  QPPQLLIYLASKLESGVPARFNGSGSGTDFTLNIHPVEEEDAATY
          QPP:LLIY AS:LESGVPARF:GSGSGTDFTLNIHPVEE:DAATY
MUVκIII   QPPKLLIYAASNLESGVPARFSGSGSGTDFTLNIHPVEEDDAATY

                   100       110
                    |         |
3α4D10Vκ  YCQQSRELPRTFGGGTKLEIK
          YCQQS.E P.TFGGGTKLEIK
MUVκIII   YCQQSNEDPXTFGGGTKLEIK
```

Alignment of (a) the VH and (b) Vκ amino acid sequences for a monoclonal antibody (3α4D10) which recognizes the toxin of *Clostridium perfringens*[52] with the consensus sequences of murine VHIIC and VκIII subfamilies. The CDRs as defined by Kabat et al[9] are underlined.

3) CDR grafting

Six synthetic oligonucleotides, each of whose sequence is the inverse complement of one of the CDRs, are constructed. Each oligonucleotide is flanked by about 12 nucleotide residues which are identical to the corresponding nucleotides in the human VH and VL genes chosen as the acceptor framework. These are annealed to the gene of the human acceptor frameworks and used to synthesize the final CDR grafted human VH and VL by asymmetric and symmetric PCR.

4) Assembly and expression of humanized antibody

The genes representing the constant domains for all human immunoglobulin subtypes have been cloned and are available. Most humanized antibodies to date have been constructed as IgG_1 or IgG_4. The VH and VL genes are cloned into a mammalian genetic engineering expression vector[10,11] and transfected into a mammalian cell line usually one of murine myeloma cell NS0, rat hybridoma YB20 or Chinese hamster ovary cells (CHO). Antibody is synthesized and secreted from such cells at levels of 2-10 μg/ml.

RESHAPING TECHNOLOGIES

Three general methods have been described and can be referred to as:

1) CDR grafting using human VH and VL frameworks with high linear amino acid sequence homology to the donor frameworks ('homology matching').[13]

2) CDR grafting using a limited subset of human frameworks selected on the basis of common usage by the human in vivo, irrespective of the linear homology between human and donor frameworks ('fixed frameworks').[14]

3) CDR grafting and computer graphic simulation of the structure of the donor murine antibody and then replacement of the murine surface amino acid residues with the most common residues found in human antibodies ('veneering').[15]

With methods 1 and 2, the current state of the art in computer graphic three dimensional modeling is inadequate to predict the conformations of CDRs and define precisely the key CDR-framework residue interactions for any one antibody. Indeed without a knowledge of the structure of the epitope of the antigen, it is unlikely that such predictions could ever be defined.

For these reasons, a number of indirect methods have been developed to assist in the selection of residue changes to be introduced into human frameworks. Comparative analysis of the X-ray structures which have been resolved has defined residues which are most likely involved in CDR-framework interactions; this definition and computer graphic modeling have together laid down a series of 'most likely' critical framework residues which are important in restoring correct conformation to CDRs which fall into particular canonical groupings.[16,17] When one analyzes the compilation of data on successfully humanized antibodies (see below) very good agreement is found between experimental and predicted results. Such predictive methodologies have greatly assisted the efficiency and quality of humanization, particularly in the last two to three years. Figure 6.4 shows a structural representation of a

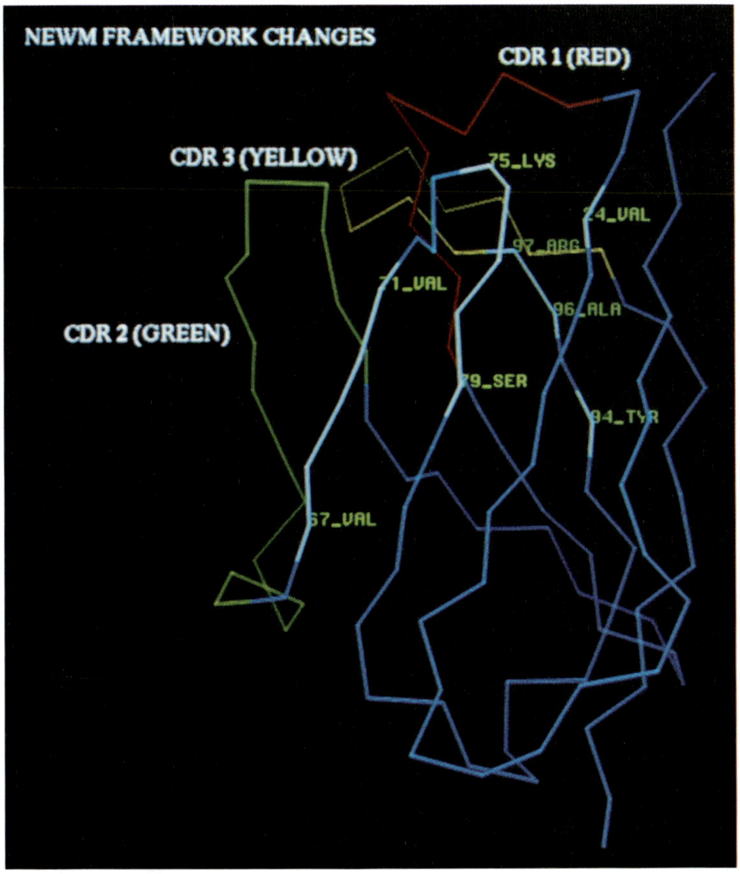

Fig. 6.4. Computer graphic model illustrating the VH framework residues most commonly involved in maintaining the conformation of CDR loops.

number of the crucial residues in VH. However, any single antibody only requires a small subset of the 'most likely' residues and their selection still requires experimentation (see later).

Homology Matching

The original methodology defined three steps:[18]

1) The VH and VL variable region amino acid sequences of the donor murine antibody are assigned to their family sub-groups and are primary sequences then compared with the consensus sequence for that sub-group. This aims to identify unusual framework amino acids which may have been introduced during in vivo maturation of the antibody producing cell and may therefore be crucial for high affinity binding of antigen. These specific residues are then earmarked for inclusion in the selected human framework.

2) VH and VL human frameworks selected on the basis of good homology to the donor are also compared with their family sub-group consensus sequences to identify unusual framework amino acids which may have been introduced during affinity maturation of the human antibody producing cell. Such residues are inferred to be required for the correct conformation of the endogenous human CDRs. Since these CDRs are being removed, then those framework residues are also replaced with the more common consensus residues.

3) Murine and human sequences are compared to eliminate consistent species differences. This method has been applied successfully to a number of antibodies.[4,8,10] An extension to this method was described by Queen and colleagues[13] whereby the linear amino acid sequence of the murine variable chains were compared directly with available human sequences and the mature human sequence with the highest homology taken as the acceptor framework.[19] This is further modified to include more commonly found human residues and in the ultimate case, synthetic consensus human frameworks are constructed.[20-23] The 'critical' murine framework residues are also then included. Some examples of humanized antibodies derived by this method are shown in Table 6.2.

Fixed Frameworks

Although there is considerable diversity in linear amino acid sequence between the framework regions of different family members of murine and human immunoglobulins, the three dimen-

Table 6.2. Representative examples of antibodies humanized by homology matching of donor murine variable region sequences with acceptor human frameworks

Human Framework	Murine Mab	No. of murine residues in addition to CDRs		References
		VH	VK	
NEWM/REI	CAMPATH-1	1	3	53
	PLAP	2	0	54
KOL/REI	OKT3	11	2	55
	CAMPATH-9	0	0	56
EU/EU	anti-Tac	12	3	57
	M195	12	6	58
	Fd138-80	11	4	59
	BMA 031	16	7	60
Consensus				
VHI/REI	mAb 425	5	1	61
VHIII/VκI	mAb 4D5	5	2	62

Table 6.3. Representative examples of antibodies humanized using fixed human frameworks VH NEWM and Vκ REI

Murine monoclonal antibody	% identity* to VHNEWM	VκREI	No. of murine residues in addition to CDRs VH	Vκ	Reference
RSV19	55	63	4	0	14
3α4D10	58	68	2	0	52
HCMV-37	66	67	5	0	63
NM01	64	67	5	1	64
VZV	59	69	6	1	65

*% identity is calculated, excluding CDRs, using 'Align Programme' of 'DNASTAR Inc.'

sional structure of the framework scaffold (Fig. 6.1) is highly conserved. There is, therefore, no a priori reason why the same human frameworks should not successfully fulfill the scaffold function of supporting CDRs derived from a broad range of donor antibodies. Table 6.3 shows a number of antibodies with widely varying linear amino acid sequence homology between donor and acceptor which have been successfully humanized using the same human frameworks NEWM and REI. These frameworks were selected on the basis that they are found commonly in vivo and have been used successfully in the clinic.

These humanized antibodies have also been developed so that there is minimal substitution of murine framework residues. Table 6.4 is a representation of the crucial framework substitutions which were required with a range of antibodies. The location of these residues within the VH structure is shown in Figure 6.4. Cumulatively humanized antibodies require the crucial framework residues identified by structural analysis and modeling. However, each individual antibody only requires a subset of these residues which may reflect the differing contributions individual CDRs make to antigen binding in different molecules. A number of humanized antibodies have been constructed to routinely include all 'critical' framework residues and are likely therefore to have more murine content than necessary (Table 6.2).

VENEERING

Since a major aim of humanization is to reduce the recognition of murine epitopes by the human immune systems, an alternate approach aims to replace exposed surface murine residues with corresponding human residues. This method, known as veneering or resurfacing,[15,24] also uses the analysis of available antibody structures to identify surface residues which are unlikely to be required for the correct conformation of hypervariable loops and can therefore be substituted with corresponding human residues. In one publication, two resurfaced antibodies, one containing 9 and the other 13 amino acid substitutions had antigen binding affinities equivalent to the progenitor murine monoclonals.[25] Such antibodies retain the interior domains of the murine antibodies but a possible disadvantage is that T cell epitopes may exist within the internal domains or be created by the interspersion of human and murine surface residues.

NEW TECHNOLOGIES IN HUMANIZING ANTIBODIES

Experience has led to improvements in methodologies for humanizing antibodies, resulting in an increased efficiency with which antigen binding affinity is restored and a reduction in the number of murine residues incorporated into human frameworks.

LOOP GRAFTING

An important realization was that the antigen binding domain represented by the hypervariable loop structures H1-H3 and L1-

Table 6.4. Representation of crucial framework substitutions required with a range of antibodies humanized using fixed VHNEWM and VHREI frameworks (Xs represent CDR residues)

```
                    10       20        30       40
                     |        |         |        |
VHNEWM      QVQLQESGPGLVRPSQTLSLTCTVSGSTFSNDY//YTWVRQPPGRG
RSHZ19      ..........................F...XXX//XX.........
3α4D10      ..............................XXX//XX.........
NM01        ..........................FSITXXXXXXX.........
VZV206      .......................A..FDFSXXX//XX.........
PS2B        .......................A......XXX//XX.........
CMV37       ...........................SITXXXX/XX.........

             50                    70       80
              |                     |        |
VHNEWM      LEWIGXXXXXXXXXXXXXXXXXRVTMLVDTSKNQFSLRLSSVTAA
RSHZ19      .....XXXXXXXXXXXXXXXX/.......................
3α4D10      .....XXXXXXXXXXXXXXXXX.......................
NM01        .....XXXXXXXXXXXXXXXX/.....R.................
VZV206      .....XXXXXXXXXXXXXXXXX.....R.................
PS2B        .....XXXXXXXXXXXXXXXXX.........SSTAY.........
CMV37       .....XXXXXXXXXXXXXXXX/.........A.............

            90      100       110
            |        |         |
VHNEWM      DTAVYYCARXXXXXXX/XXXWGQGTTVTVSS
RSHZ19      .....F.NSXXXX////XXX...........
3α4D10      .......NAXXXXXX/XXXX...........
NM01        .........XXXXXXXXXXX...........
VZV206      .........XXXXXXX///X...........
PS2B        .........XXXXXXXXX/X...........
CMV37       .....F...XXXXXXXX///...........
```

L3 (chapter 1) do not strictly accord with CDRs as identified from linear sequence homology. Commonly, for example, structural analysis places VH amino acid residues 26-32 within H-1 while, by the definition of Kabat and colleagues, CDR-1 is designated as residues 31-35. 'Loop grafting' is, therefore, more appropriate as the first step in humanizing an antibody. If loop grafting had been carried out initially with the antibodies described in Table 6.4, residues 27-30 would have been included. It can be seen that in 3/6 of the antibodies these residues were crucial for restoration of antigen binding.

The elucidation of the sequence of essentially all the human VH and Vκ germ line segments has resulted in the categorization of 5 of the 6 hypervariable loops into a small number of main chain conformations (canonical structures) which are largely common between mouse and human[26] providing the opportunity to transfer antigen binding affinity by grafting only parts of murine loops or key murine residues into partially preserved human hypervariable loops.

Germ Line Frameworks

The selection of VH and VL human frameworks as the acceptor molecules for humanized antibodies has to date been made from the extensive data base of human antibody sequences derived from adult myeloma or lymphoblastoid cell lines. The great majority of such antibodies contain somatic mutations introduced during in vivo affinity maturation into the CDRs and/or framework regions of the progenitor germ line genes in the pre-B cell. Adult antibodies can contain 8-15 somatic mutations. While a few of these are directly concerned with increasing antigen binding affinity, many are background noise arising from random mutation. The individual within whom such mutations arise has the opportunity to develop tolerance to such altered molecules, but the population in general do not. There is the possibility, therefore, that such somatic mutations can give rise to immunogenic epitopes. Recent years have seen the elucidation of the nucleotide and amino acid sequences of virtually all the human VH and VL germ line repertoire.[27-30] It is now possible, therefore, to select human germ line VH and VL as acceptors for humanization and thereby eliminate the small potential for immunogenicity of adult VH and VL.[31] Table 6.5 compares the adult VH NEWM and VL REI with the most likely germ line progenitors. It can be seen that the adult antibodies contain 10 somatic mutations for VH and 5 for VL respectively. The murine monoclonal antibody 3α4D10 which binds to the α-toxin of *Clostridium perfringens* was humanized by the fixed framework methodology using adult NEWM and REI as acceptor human frameworks.[52] Subsequently, mutations have been introduced to convert the frameworks back to their germ line equivalents. Figure 6.5 compares the antigen binding affinity of 'adult' and 'germ-line' humanized 3α4D10 from which it can be seen that humanized antibodies can equally well be provided using human germ line frameworks.

Table 6.5. HUVH(NEWM) and HUVκ(REI) adult sequences aligned with their germ line equivalents and Mab 3α4D10 humanized with human germ lines

(a) VHNEWM ADULT FRAMEWORK
(b) VHNEWM GERM-LINE FRAMEWORK(hvh4go16)
(c) 3α4D10/VHNEWM GERM-LINE FRAMEWORK
(d) VκREI ADULT FRAMEWORK
(e) VκREI GERM-LINE FRAMEWORK(lvh3g26)
(f) 3α4D10/VKREI GERM-LINE FRAMEWORK

```
VHNEWM
                *  *      *             *     *
(a) QVQLQESGPGLVRPSQTLSLTCTVSGSTFSXXXXXWVRQPPGRG
(b) ............K..D......A.............I.....K.
(c) ............K..D......A.......XXXXX.I.....K.

                              *          *      *
(a) LEWIGXXXXXXXXXXXXXXXXXRVTMLVDTSKNQFSLRLSSVTAA
(b) ..........................S..........K......V
(c) .....XXXXXXXXXXXXXXXXX....S..........K......V

                         *  *
(a) DTAVYYCARXXXXXXXXXXWGQTTVTVSS
(b) .....................K..L....
(c) .......NAXXXXXXXXXX..K..L....

VκREI
       *                               *
(d) DIQLTQSPSSLSASVGDRVTITCXXXXXXXXXXXWYQQKPGKAP
(e) ...M...................XXXXXXXXXXX.F........
(f) ...M...................XXXXXXXXXXX.F........

                               *         *
(d) KLLIYXXXXXXGVPSRFSGSGSGTDFTFTISSLQPEDIATYYC
(e) ...........................L.........F.....
(f) .....XXXXXXX...............L.........F.....

                  *
(d) XXXXXXXXXFGQTKVEIKRE
(e) XXXXXXXXX.....L.....
(f) XXXXXXXXX.....L.....
```

ALLOTYPIC VARIANTS

The human population has polymorphic determinants in the constant region, VH and VL and a therapeutic antibody of one allotype may be immunogenic in that proportion of the population with different allotypes. This concept has been discussed in detail previously.[32,33] In the constant region of IgG there are 17

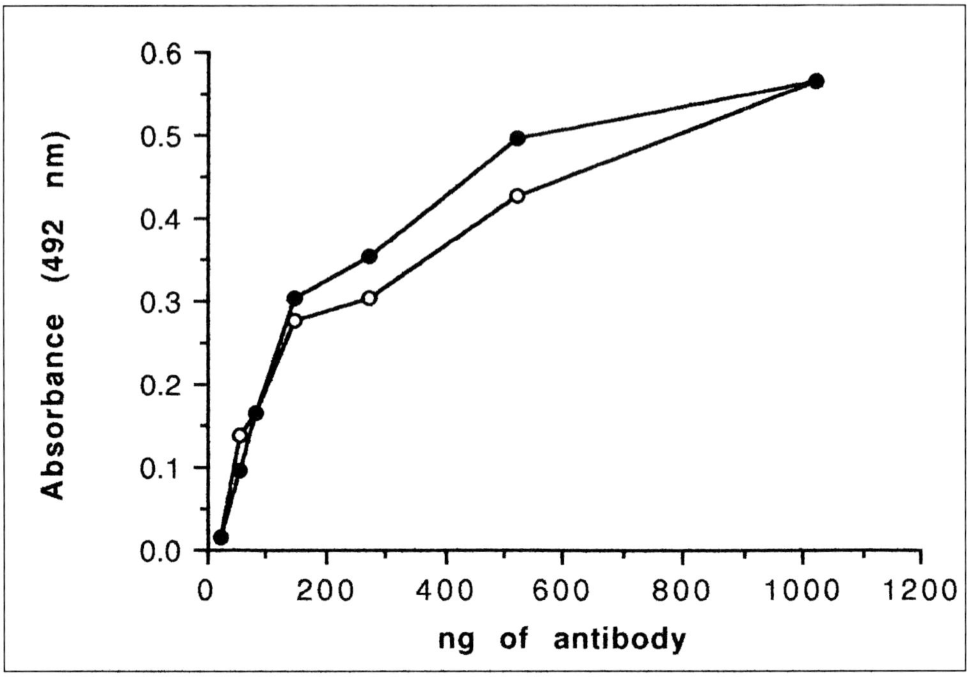

Fig. 6.5. ELISA assay comparing the relative binding to phospholipase C of 3α4D10 humanized (●) and germ line equivalent (O) antibodies. Data of Emery S & Harris WJ (unpublished).

allotypes observed with reasonable frequency in the population: IgG_1 has 4, IgG_2 has 1, IgG_3 has 13 and IgG_4 has none. There are allotypes of human heavy and κ light chains. It may be appropriate then to select the most frequent allotypes in the population and accept that some patients may be able to react to allotypic differences. For example, the allele G1m(1) is most common constant region allotype in the European population and VH germ line DP49 (VH1111) has been found to be identical in 92% of 52 individuals suggesting there is little allotypic variation.[33]

Undesirable Human Framework Regions

The in vivo use of human frameworks is not random, suggesting that some frameworks may be more appropriate for inclusion in therapeutic antibodies than others, particularly since during therapy these frameworks will be present in the body in concentrations much higher than in nature. There is very little information available on the biological implications and activities of different frameworks and framework combinations which would allow selection at the present time. However, it is known that all cold agglutinins are derived from the VH4-21 gene.[34] It would seem expedient then to avoid choosing this framework for a therapeutic.

PRECLINICAL STUDIES WITH HUMANIZED ANTIBODIES

Table 6.6 describes results of in vivo studies of humanized antibodies in primates. Data derived from primate studies offers a valuable insight into likely clinical behavior. As discussed in chapter 4, such studies with chimeric antibodies have shown improved pharmacokinetics and reduced immunogenicity compared with rodent antibodies and the cumulative data from humanized antibodies has confirmed this trend (Table 6.6).

When primates were treated with multiple doses of murine anti-Tac (0.05 mg/kg - 5.0 mg/kg), all animals developed an immune response against the variable and constant regions of the antibody resulting in rapid plasma clearance. By contrast, the immune response to humanized anti-Tac was 5-10-fold less, occurred only in a subset of animals and was anti-idiotypic only.[35] No antibody response was detected in primates treated with up to 5 mg/kg of HuM195. Similarly, the antibody response against humanized CDP571 (anti-TNFα) was less than 5% of that recorded with the murine antibody.[37] In the most extensive studies, no antibody response was detected in cynomologous monkeys even when given up to 50 mg/kg of humanized anti-RSV, a dose many fold in excess of likely therapeutic regimes.[38]

Table 6.6. Humanized antibodies in cynomologous monkeys

Antibody	Doses (mg/kg)	t1/2β	HAMA
Humanized			
Anti-Tac	0.05-5.0	100-200 hours	?
Anti-TNFα	0.05-1.0	72 hours	0/4
M-195	0.05-5.0	14 days	0/3
Anti-RSV	1.0-50.0	16-21 days	0/4
Human			
C23 (anti-HCMV)	20.0	20 days	-
Ev-27	0.5-16.0	18 days	1/5
Murine	1.0-10.0	20-50 hours	100%

See text for references

Serum half-lives with humanized antibodies are similar to those one would expect from human antibodies in primates (Table 6.6) and in the absence of target antigen reach 14-21 days. Table 6.6 includes data with human monoclonals[39] for comparison and shows that the behavior of humanized and human monoclonals in primates is equivalent

CLINICAL STUDIES WITH HUMANIZED ANTIBODIES

Table 6.7 shows those humanized antibodies currently in clinical trial.

CAMPATH-1H

CAMPATH-1H has been studied in a number of small trials to deplete lymphocytes either alone or in combination with a non-depleting anti-CD4 monoclonal to block the function of T helper cells. In a study of four patients with rheumatoid arthritis, mild fever, rigors and nausea were noted shortly after the first infusion. These symptoms were thought to be due to lympholysis mediated by the release of cytokines. Good depletion of $CD40^+$ lymphocytes was obtained with cells returning only 90 days after a single dose. Significant clinical benefits and short term remissions were observed in all patients.[40] Repeated treatment with CAMPATH-1H was effective though some patients eventually developed an anti-idiotype response. In further studies, remissions from symptoms of rheumatoid arthritis have been maintained for 120-360 days.

Table 6.7. Humanized antibodies in clinical trial

Antibody	t1/2β	HAMA
Humanized		
CAMPATH-1	-	0/8, 3/4
Anti-PLAP	68 hours	0/7
Anti-Tac	4 days	0/12
M-195	23-54 hours	0/13
Anti-TNFα	7-14 days	0/6
Anti-RSV	++++++++	0
Human		
Anti-CMV	13-17days	0

See text for references

Successful clearance of malignant cells from the blood and bone marrow in two patients with non-Hodgkin's B cell lymphoma was achieved since much higher concentrations of antibodies (126 mg over 30 days and 86 mg over 43 days) were tolerated than previously possible with the progenitor rat antibody. One patient relapsed four months after the first course of antibody treatment but a second course of 65 mg over 12 days again eliminated the malignant cells and provided 15 months remission.[41] A phase I/II trial in non-Hodgkin's lymphoma and chronic lymphocytic leukemia showed positive clinical responses with a low level of HAMA response in a small percentage of patients.[42] CAMPATH-1H, with or without additional anti-CD4 antibody, has shown that long term remissions in patients with vasculitis can be achieved with short term therapy.[43] Results in six patients with progressive multiple sclerosis have been very encouraging. Prior to treatment, patients cumulatively possessed 27 brain plaque lesions as detected by MRI. Only two lesions had returned nine months after the single dose.[44] Formal phase II trials are being carried out by Wellcome plc.

Anti-Interleukin-2 Receptor

Anti-Tac (T cell activation antigen) is a humanized IgG_1 monoclonal antibody directed against the α chain (p55) of the human IL-2 receptor on activated T-lymphocytes. The antibody was humanized by homology matching and contains a considerable number of murine residues in addition to the CDRs (Table 6.2).

In the initial phase I trials conducted by Hoffman-La Roche, single doses of 0.5, 1.0 or 1.5 mg/kg were administered to 20 bone marrow transplant patients with steroid resistant graft-versus-host disease (GVHD).[45] There were no appreciable side effects. Overall improvement of GVHD occurred in eight patients with four complete and four partial responses. Positive clinical responses were also seen with three key markers for GVHD: skin disease (9/16), liver disease (3/15) and gastrointestinal disease (6/12). Two patients have survived 18-21 months. Pharmacokinetics showed a terminal elimination half-life of four days which is similar to that reported for human immunoglobulins administered in the post-transplant period (5-10 days). There was no HAMA response reported in any patients in contrast to earlier studies with murine anti-IL2R where a HAMA response was found in 4/8 patients. A multinational phase II/III trial began in April 1993 with multiple doses for the prevention of GVHD. Data from this study are expected in mid-1995. A phase I study of patients receiving kidney transplants is also ongoing.

ANTI-CD33

Murine antibody M195 is directed against CD33 antigen present on leukemia cells of most patients with acute (AML) or chronic (CML) myeloid leukemia but is absent from hematopoetic stem cells. When administered as an ^{131}I radioimmunoconjugate, the murine monoclonal effectively reduced the number of peripheral blood and bone marrow blast cells in patients with relapsed or refractory AML but 7/17 patients developed HAMA which prevented further treatment. A phase I trial of humanized M195 (HuM195, IgG_1; Table 6.7) involved 13 patients receiving 6 doses of 0.5, 1.0, 3.0 or 10.0 mg/m^2 over a period of 18 days.[46] Two patients received a second dosing regime of 12 doses (cumulatively 216 mg of HuM195). The first dose was trace-labeled with ^{131}I to follow pharmacokinetics. The entire bone marrow was specifically and clearly imaged with optimal biodistribution at 3 mg/m^2 level. Absorption to targeted sites of disease was observed and the antibody was well tolerated with only the patients receiving 10 mg/m^2 experiencing adverse effects in the form of grade 2 fever and grade 2 rigors in 2/3 cases; these effects were prevented by pre-medication with diphenhydramine and acetominophen. No HAMA response was found, even after 19 weeks and 6-12 doses of therapy. This is in contrast to the above report with the murine antibody. Plasma and whole body half lives were 38 and 51 hours which was similar to that found with murine M195. This short half life is likely to be due to constant production and renewal of CD33 containing leukemia cells binding all available antibody.

ANTI-TNFα RECEPTOR

A phase I trial in human healthy volunteers of the anti-TNF antibody CDP571 used single doses of 0.1 mg/kg, 0.3 mg/kg, 1.0 mg/kg, 5.0 mg/kg and 10.0 mg/kg.[47] All doses were well tolerated and a mean $t1/2\beta$ of 13 days was observed (range 4-22 days). A small temporary anti-CDP571 IgM response was observed 2-3 weeks after dosing but had declined by 6 weeks. However, the highest HAMA response was obtained with the lowest doses of 0.1 mg/kg and 0.3 mg/kg with no detectable HAMA response at doses greater than 2.0 mg/kg. This small HAMA response did not significantly affect antibody binding to TNFα or CDP571 clearance.

ANTI-RESPIRATORY SYNCYTIAL VIRUS

SB 209763 is a humanized IgG_1 antibody derived from the murine antibody RSV19 directed to the fusion (F) protein of respiratory syncytial virus (RSV).[14] It has been shown to rapidly clear RSV infections from the pulmonary tract of mice, cotton rats and cattle.[48-50] Primate studies have demonstrated safety and long half-life of 21 days even at intravenous doses of up to 200 mg/kg[38] which is many fold in excess of likely therapeutic doses. A phase I trial in healthy volunteers was completed in 1994 and initial analysis has demonstrated safety, extended half-life and no HAMA response. A phase II trial in children under two years old with RSV infection is ongoing.

PRIMATIZED ANTIBODIES

A novel approach based upon the use of a monoclonal antibody recovered from immunized monkeys has been applied to develop a primatized anti-CD4 monkey-human IgG_1 chimeric.[51] This antibody, which blocks CD4 antigen on helper T cells, has been used in a phase I study of 25 patients with moderate-severe rheumatoid arthritis. No toxicity was observed during a single intravenous dosing regime from 0.03 mg/kg to 4.0 mg/kg, nor was any immune response detectable in any patient. There was evidence for clinical improvement in 13/25 patients. A multi-dose phase I/II trial is ongoing.

FUTURE PROSPECTS WITH HUMANIZED ANTIBODIES

Over 80 humanized antibodies have been described[3] which target a broad range of antigens for the treatment of cancer, infections, autoimmune disease, immunosuppression and tolerance. A representative listing of those with good therapeutic potential is shown in Table 6.8. It is likely that about 20 will have moved into clinical trial by the end of 1995 and many more in 1996. This is, therefore, a well established product range.

Current limited data have confirmed their safety, extended half-life, and minimal HAMA response compared to murine and chimeric monoclonals. The inclusion of human effector functions has increased the potency over murine counterparts where complement

Table 6.8. Representative examples of humanized antibodies with therapeutic potential

Antibody	Antigen	Therapy	Company	Current Status	Ref.
Anti-infectives					
RSHZ19	F-protein	Respiratory syncytial virus	Scotgen/ Smith-Beecham	Phase II	14
HCMV-16	gH-protein	Human cytomegalovirus	Scotgen/ Biopharmaceuticals	Pre-clinical	66
CMV-5	gH protein	Human cytomegalovirus	Protein Design Laboratories	Pre-clinical	39
Fd138-80	gD protein	Herpes simplex virus-1	Protein Design Labs	Pre-clinical	59
NM-01	gP-120	Human Immunodeficiency Virus	Scotgen/ Nissin Research Institute	Pre-clinical	64
Tumor Antigens					
4D5	$P\text{-}185^{HER2}$	Breast Cancer	Genentech	Phase I/II	62
B72-3	TAG-72		Celltech/American Cynamid	Research	67
CDP671	Human milk fat globulin		Celltech/American Cynamid	Phase I	68
A5B7	CEA	Colon Cancer	Celltech	Pre-clinical	69
425	EGFR		MRC Collaborative Center/E Merk	Pre-clinical	61
ABL364	Lewis Y Antigen		Protein Design Labs/Sandoz	Pre-clinical	70
M195	CD33	CML	Protein Design Labs	Phase I/II	46
35/93	Lewis Y	Colon	LICR/Scotgen	Pre-clinical	77
BW431/26	CEA		Behring werke	Pre-clinical	10
CAMPATH-1H		NHL	Wellcome Plc	Phase III	42
Immunosuppression					
OKT3	CD4	Transplantation	Celltech/RW. Johnson Prl	Pre-clinical	55
OKT 4A	CD4		Celltech/RW. Johnson Prl	Pre-clinical	71
CAMPATH-9	CD4		Cambridge Pathology	Pre-clinical	56
ANTI-TAC	CD25	GVHD	Protein Design Laboratories/Hoffman La Roche	Phase II	45
CAMPATH-6	CD25	GVHD	Wellcome Foundation	Phase I/II	72
CDP571	TNF-α		Celltech/Bayer	Phase I/II	47
Autoimmune Disease					
HP 1/2	CD49a		Scotgen/Biogen	Pre-clinical	73
022	CD64		Scotgen/Medarex	Phase I	74
CAMPATH-9	CD4	Rheumatoid Arthritis	Cambridge Pathology	Pre-clinical	56
TM23	TCR 5.2/5.3	Multiple Sclerosis	Scotgen/T Cell Sciences	Pre-clinical	60
BMA031	TCR$\alpha\beta$		Behringwerke	Research	75
CAMPATH-1		Rheumatoid Arthritis/ Multiple Sclerosis	Wellcome Foundation	Phase I	40/44
Cardiovascular					
C4G1	CD41a (GPIIb/IIIa)	Atherosclerosis	Protein Design Labs/ Yamanouchi	Pre-clinical	76

or ADCC directed cytotoxicity are invoked.[4] As part of product development programs, mammalian cells are developed which, in large scale fermentation, can provide greater than 1 g\L of humanized antibody. These antibodies can therefore be used cost effectively in large doses and regimes of several hundred milligrams per dose can be contemplated. This contrasts with available human antibodies derived from EBV transformed lymphoblastoid cell lines or heterohybridomas where yields from cell culture are severely limiting dosing regimes in clinical studies. For prophylactic or chronic treatment, monthly doses with humanized antibodies should suffice to maintain very high serum titers.

Humanized antibodies, therefore, represent a new class of therapeutics. In cancer treatment, it is possible for the first time to evaluate the ability of a fully recruited human immune defense system to deplete cancer cells over extended periods of time. There is a promising opportunity for chronic treatment of autoimmune diseases with the exciting potential that short term therapy by interfering with immunoregulatory controls may give rise to long term remission. In infectious diseases, neutralizing humanized monoclonal antibodies with several thousand-fold more potency than hyperimmune polyclonal sera offer the opportunity for efficacy comparable to traditional drugs with the added value of long term passive protection.

References

1. Jones PT, Dear PH, Foote J et al. Replacing the complementary determining regions in a human antibody with those from a mouse. Nature 1986; 321:522-525.
2. Winter G, Harris WJ. Humanized antibodies. Immunol Today 1993; 14:243-246.
3. Emery S, Adair JR. Humanised monoclonal antibodies for therapeutic applications. Exp Opin Invest Drugs 1994; 3:241-251.
4. Mountain A, Adair JR. Engineering antibodies for therapy. Biotech Gen Eng Rev 1992; 10:1-142.
5. Clark M. Protein Engineering of Antibody Molecules for Prophylactic and Therapeutic Applications in Man. London: Academic Press, 1993.
6. Wright A, Shin SU, Morrison SL. Genetically engineered antibodies: progress and prospects. Crit Rev Immunol 1992; 12:125-168.
7. Adair J. Engineering antibodies for therapy. Immunol Rev 1992; 130:5-40.
8. Harris WJ. Humanizing monolonal antibodies for *in vivo* use. In: Spiers RE, Griffiths JB, eds. Animal Cell Biotechnology. London: Academic Press, 1994; 6:259-279.

9. Kabat EA, Wu TT, Reid-Miller M et al. Sequences of Proteins of Immunological Interest. 5th ed. Bethesda: United States Department of Health and Human Services, 1991.
10. Gussow D, Seeman G. Humanisation of monoclonal antibodies. Methods Emzymol. 1991; 203:99-121.
11. Emery SC, Harris WJ. Strategies for humanising antibodies. In: Borrebaeck CAK, ed. Antibody Engineering: A Practical Guide. New York: Oxford University Press, (in press).
12. Orlandi R, Gussow DH, Jones PT et al. Cloning immunoglobulin variable domains for expression by the polymerase chain reaction. Proc Nat Acad Sci 1989; 86:3833-3837.
13. Queen C, Schneider WP, Selick HE et al. A humanised antibody that binds to the interleukin 2 receptor. Proc Nat Acad Sci 1989; 86:10029-10033.
14. Tempest PR, Bremner P, Lambert M et al. Reshaping a human monoclonal antibody to inhibit respiratory syncytial virus infection *in vivo*. Biotechnology 1991; 9:266-271.
15. Padlan EA. A possible procedure for reducing the immunogenicity of antibody variable domains while preserving their ligand binding properties. Mol Immunol 1991; 28:489-498.
16. Foote J, Winter G. Antibody framework residues affecting the conformation of hypervariable loops. J Mol Biol 1992; 224:487-499.
17. Chothia C, Lesk AM, Tramontano A et al. Conformations of imunoglobulin hypervariable regions. Nature 1989; 342:877-883.
18. Verhoeyen M, Milstein C, Winter G. Reshaping human antibodies: grafting an anti-lysozyme activity. Science 1988; 239:1098-1104.
19. Singer IJ, Kawka DW, deMartino JA et al. Optimal humanisation of 1B4, an anti-CD-18 murine monoclonal antibody is achieved by correct choice of human V-region framework sequences. J Immunol 1993; 150:2844-2857.
20. Co M, Deschamps M, Whitley RJ et al. Humanised antibodies for antiviral therapy. Proc Nat Acad Sci 1991; 88:2869-2873.
21. Maeda H, Matsushita S, Eda Y et al. Construction of reshaped human antibodies with HIV neutralising activity. Human Antibody Hybridomas 1991; 2:124-134.
22. Presta LG, Lahr SJ, Shields RL et al. Humanization of an antibody directed against IgE. J Immunol 1993; 151:2623-2632.
23. Kolbinger F, Saldanha J, Hardman N et al. Humanisation of a mouse anti-human IgE antibody: a potential therapeutic for IgE mediated allergies. Protein Eng 1993; 6:971-980.
24. Pederson JT, Henry AH, Searle SJ et al. Comparison of surface accessible residues in human and murine immunoglobulin Fv domains. J Mol Biol 1994; 235:959-973.
25. Roguska MA, Pederson JT, Keddy CA et al. Humanisation of murine monoclonal antibodies through variable domain resurfacing. Proc Nat Acad Sci 1994; 91:969-973.

26. Chothia C, Lesk AM, Gerardi E et al. Structural repertoire of the human VH segments. J Mol Biol 1992; 227:799-817
27. Tomlinson IM, Walter G, Marks JD et al. The repertoire of human germ line VH sequences reveals about 50 groups of VH segments with different hypevariable loops. J Mol Biol 1992; 227:776-798.
28. Matsuda F, Shin EK, Naguoka H et al. Structure and physical map of 64 variable segments in the 3' 0.8-megabase region of the human immunoglobulin heavy chain locus. Nature Genet 1993; 3:88-94.
29. Schable KF, Zachau H-G. The variable genes of the human immunoglobulin κ locus. Biol Chem Hoppe-Seyler 1993; 374: 1001-1022.
30. Cook G, Tomlinson IM, Walter G et al. A map of the human immunoglobulin VH locus completed by analysis of the telomeric region of chromosome 14q. Nature Genet 1994; 7:162-168.
31. Winter GP, Carr FJ, Harris WJ. Altered antibodies; products and processes relating thereto. 1993. Patent WO93/17105.
32. Gorman SD, Clark MR. Humanisation of monoclonal antibodies for therapy. Sem Immunol 1990; 2:457-466.
33. Routledge EG, Gorman SD, Clark M. In: Clark M, ed. Protein Engineering of Antibody Molecules for Prophylactic and Therapeutic Applications in Man. London: Academic Press, 1993:13-44.
34. Pascual V, Victor K, Lelsz D et al. Nucleotide sequence analysis of the V regions of two IgM cold agglutinins. Evidence that the VH 4-21 gene segment is responsible for the major cross-reactive idiotpye. J Immunol 1991; 146:4385-4391.
35. Hakimi J, Chizzonite R, Luke D et al. Reduced immunogenciity and improved pharmacokinetics of humanised anti-Tac in cynomologous monkeys. J Immunol 1991; 147:1352-1359.
36. Cornett J. Pharmacokinetics and immunogenicity of human and humanized monoclonal antibodies: implications for therapy. Proc IBC Conference, Antibody Based Therapeutics, Washington, DC 1994.
37. Stephens S. Clinical studies with the recombinant anti-TNF antibody CDP571. Proc IBC Conf: Antibody Engineering, Coronado, 1993.
38. Hart TK, Ruggieri EV, Demuth SG et al. Antigenicity of RSHZ19, a reshaped human antibody, in cynomologous Macaques following a single intravenous administration. Proc IBC Conference; Antibody Based Therapeutics, Washington DC, 1994.
39. Nadler P, Wood DL, Ostberg L et al. The use of human and genetically engineered humanized antibodies for the prophylaxis and treatment of cytomegalovirus infection. Transplant Immunol Lett 1994; IX:5-15.
40. Isaacs JD, Watts RA, Hazleman BL et al. Humanised monoclonal antibody therapy for rheumatoid arthritis. Lancet 1992; 340: 748-752.

41. Hale G, Dyer MJ, Clark MR et al. Remission induction in non-Hodgkin's lymphoma with reshaped human monoclonal antibody CAMPATH-1H. Lancet 1988; ii:1394-1399.
42. Lim SH, Hale G, Marcos RE et al. CAMPATH-1 monoclonal antibody therapy in severe refractory autoimmune thrombocytopenic purura. Br J Haematol 1993; 84:542-4.
43. Lockwood CM, Thiru S, Isaacs JD et al. Humanised monoclonal antibody treatment for intractable systemic vasculitis. Lancet 1993; 341: 620-1622.
44. Hale G. unpublished data.
45. Anasetti C, Hansen JA, Waldmann TA et al. Treatment of acute graft-versus-host disease with humanised anti-Tac: an antibody that binds to the interleukin-2 receptor. Blood 1994; 84:1320-1327.
46. Caron PC, Jurcic JG, Scott AM et al. A phase IB trial of humanised monoclonal antibody M195 (anti-CD33) in myeloid leukemia: specific targeting without immunogenicity. Blood 1994; 83:1760-1768.
47. Bodmer M. Monoclonal antibodies recognising cytokines. IIR Conf: *In vivo* use of Monoclonal Antibodies, London, 1993.
48. Stott EJ, Taylor G. In: Dimmock NJ, Minor PD, eds. Immune Responses, Virus Infections and Disease. London: IRL Press, 1989:85-104.
49. Taylor G, Stott EJ, Bew M et al. Monoclonal antibodies protect against respiratory syncytial virus infection in mice. Immunology 1983; 52:137-142.
50. Taylor G, Furze J, Tempest PR et al. Humanised monoclonal antibody to respiratory syncytial virus. Lancet 1991; 337:1411-1412.
51. Solinger AM. First clinical trial with a primatized monoclonal anti-CD4 antibody. Proc IBC Conference Antibody Engineering, San Diego, 1994; Vol.2.
52. Tempest PR, White P, Williamson ED et al. Efficient generation of a reshaped human mAb specific for the α-toxin of *Clostridium perfringens*. Protein Eng 1991; 7:1501-1507.
53. Reichmann NL, Clark M, Waldmann H et al. Reshaping human antibodies for therapy. Nature 1988; 332:323-327.
54. Verhoeyen M, Broderick L, Eida S et al. Reshaped human anti-PLAP antibodies. In: Epenetos AA, ed. Monoclonal Antibodies: Applications in Clinical Oncology. Chapman and Hall Medical: UK. 1991:37-43.
55. Woodle ES, Thistlewaite JR, Jolliffe LK et al. Humanised OKT-3 antibodies: successful transfer of immune modulating properties and idiotype expression. J Immunol 1992; 148:2756-2763.
56. Gorman SD, Clark MR, Routledge EG et al. Reshaping a therapeutic CD4 antibody. Proc Nat Acad Sci 1991; 88:4181-4185.
57. Brown PS, Parenteau GL, Dirbas FM et al. Anti-Tac-H. A humanised antibody to the interleukin-2 receptor. Proc Nat Acad Sci 1991; 88:2663-2667.

58. Co MS, Avdalovic NM, Caron PC et al. Chimeric and humanised antibodies with specificity for the CD33 antigen. J Immunol 1992; 148:1149-1154.
59. Co MS, Deschamps M, Whitley RJ et al. Humanised antibodies for antiviral therapy. Proc Nat Acad Sci 1991; 88:2869-2873.
60. Shearman CW, Pollock D, White G et al. Construction, expression and characterisation of humanized antibodies directed against the human alpha/beta T cell receptor. J Immunol 1991; 147: 4366-4373.
61. Kettleborough CA, Saldanha J, Heath VJ et al. Humanisation of a mouse monoclonal antibody by CDR grafting. The importance of framework residues on loop conformation. Protein Eng 1991; 4:773-783.
62. Carter P, Presta L, Gorman CM et al. Humanization of an anti-p185 Her2 antibody for human cancer therapy. Proc Nat Acad Sci 1992; 89:4285-4289.
63. Tempest PR, White P, Buttle M et al. Identification of framework residues required to restore antigen binding during reshaping of a monoclonal antibody against the glycoprotein gB of human cytomegalovirus. Int J Biol Macromolecules, (in press).
64. Nakamura A, Sasaki H, Terada M et al. Complement-dependent virolysis of HIV-1 with monoclonal antibody NM-01. AIDS Research and Human Retroviruses. 1993; 9:619-626.
65. Moss M, Grose C, Carr F et al. Reshaping of an anti-varicella zoster virus antibody. 2nd International Conference on the Varicella Zoster Virus, Paris, 1994.
66. Grundy JE, Hamilton A, Roy DM et al. A humanised cytomegalovirus specific monoclonal antibody for prophylaxis and therapy. Int Conf: Infections of the Immunocompromised Host, Davis, 1994.
67. Adair JR, Athwal DS, Emtage JS. Humanised Antibodies. 1991. Patent WO91/09967
68. Adair JR, Owens RJ, Baker TS et al. Anti-human milk fat globulin antibodies, 1993. Patent WO 93/06231.
69. Adair JR, Bodmer MW, Mountain A et al. CDR Grafted anti-CEA antibodies and their production, 1992. Patent WO92/01059.
70. Co MS, Loibner H. Antibody derivatives, 1993. Patent EP 0528767 A1.
71. Jolliffee LK, Zivin RA, Pulito VL et al. CDR grafted antibodies, 1991. Patent WO91/09966.
72. Waldmann H, Winter GP, Crowe JS et al. Humanised interleukin-2 receptor antibodies. 1993. Patent WO93/01289.
73. Leone DR, Tempest PR, White PR et al. Humanisation of an anti-$\alpha 4$ integrin monoclonal antibody for human therapy (in press).
74. Fanger MW, Segal DM, Romet-Lemonne J-L. Bispecific antibodies and targeted cellular cytotoxicity. Immunol Today 1991; 12:51-54.

75. Lin A, Stewart S, Henry L et al. Humanisation and expression of a monoclonal antibody specific to human TCRβ5.2 and 5.3 T cells. 4th Annual IBC International Conference on Antibody Engineering, San Diego, 1993.
76. Co MS, Yano S, Hsu RK et al. A humanised monoclonal antibody specific for the platelet integrin gpIIb/IIIa. J Immunol 1994; 152:2968-2976.
77. Kitamura K, Stockert E, Garin-Chesa P et al. Specificity analysis of blood group Lewis-Y (Ley) antibodies generated against synthetic and natural Ley determinants. Proc Nat Acad Sci 1994; 91: 12957-12961.

CHAPTER 7

Bacteriophage Antibody Display Libraries

INTRODUCTION

Human monoclonal antibodies remain difficult to make by immortalization of B cells and even if this technology is ultimately perfected, it will be particularly difficult to isolate human monoclonal antibodies against human (self) antigens unless the antigen is 'fortuitously' a target in autoimmune disease. This occurs because the human body rapidly develops tolerance and eliminates B cells expressing antibodies against self antigens.

The display of the human immunoglobulin repertoire on filamentous phage has provided a major new approach to providing human antibodies against a broad range of antigens including self antigens and the technology is likely to be a fruitful source of therapeutics in the next 5-10 years.

BACKGROUND

The diverse libraries of high affinity antibodies found in vivo are derived by two main processes:

1) The assembly of VH and VL domains by a combinatorial process from genetic elements in the germ line. This generates a human pre-B cell population of about 10^{12} cells displaying on their surfaces naive antibodies of low affinity (10^{-6} to 10^{-7} M). Antigen binding to the pre-B cell stimulates cell proliferation and thus preferential selection of a cell population displaying antibody against

the presented antigen. Antigen recognition of antibody is likely to be on the basis of overall shape complementarity between antigen and antibody and binding affinity between antigen and CDR3-H and CDR3-L.[1]

2) Antigen-driven pre-B cell proliferation is accompanied by somatic mutation within VH and Vκ\λ gene segments resulting in the selection of antibody-producing cells with higher binding affinity for antigen (10^{-8} to 10^{-9} M). Somatic mutations in either CDR or framework residues modify the antigen binding surface so that specific interactions between antigen and antibody are strengthened, principally through increased bonding with CDR1-H and CDR1-L or CDR2-H and CDR2-L.[2]

It is these processes that have been mimicked in vitro to generate combinatorial antibody libraries by making use of the polymerase chain reaction to amplify VH and VL genetic populations and to assemble Fab and Fv fragments of immunoglobulins in *E. coli.*[3-6]

CONSTRUCTION OF HUMAN BACTERIOPHAGE LIBRARIES

Bacteriophage Hosts

The methodology for the construction of a human bacteriophage library is show in Figure 7.1. The repertoire of antibody VH and VL genes can be recovered from peripheral blood lymphocytes, spleen or tonsils by PCR and cloned in-frame into the capsid gene of bacteriophages such as Fd and M13 and displayed on the surface of phage particles.[6,7] The antibody, displayed as either a ScFv, Fd or Fab fusion product retains the structure of the antigen binding domain and can thus be bound by antigen. Antigen can then be used to separate the desired phage from the combinatorial library. As the filamentous particle contains a single stranded copy of the phage genome, selection of the antibody also results in selection of the gene encoding that antibody. The process thereby mimics pre-B cell selection as described above.

A variety of formats are available for phage display[8] including cloning directly into filamentous coliphages such as Fd or plasmid based phagemid vectors. In phage display, antibody can be fused to either the minor capsid protein pIII to display 3-5 copies of antibody per phage particle[9,10] or to the major capsid protein pVIII

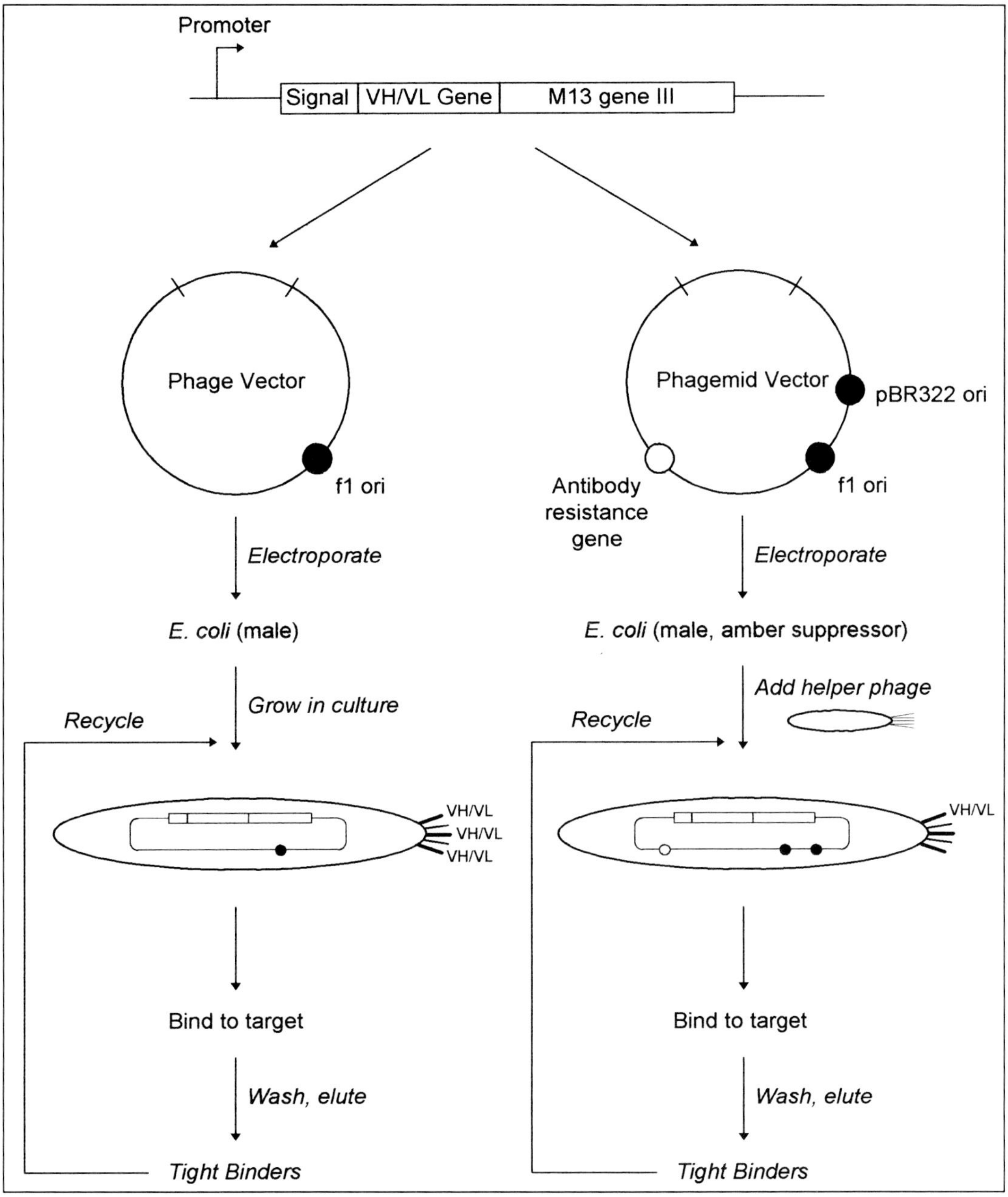

Fig. 7.1. Schematic representation of construction and selection of bacteriophage displaying antibody fragments. VH/VL genes are fused to M13 gene III in either phage or phagemid vector format and grown in E. coli. *Phage binding to antigen are selected by immunoaffinity absorption to antigen and subjected to several rounds of selection. Reproduced with permission from: Clackson T, James A.* In vitro *selection from protein and peptide libraries. Trends Biotech 1994; 12:173-184; © Elsevier Trends in Journals, Cambridge.*

to display about 2700 antibody fragments per phage particle.[11] An amber codon can be inserted into the gene at the junction of the antibody and capsid protein to allow the option of producing unfused antibody in a soluble form by transfecting phage into supE$^-$ *E. coli*. The fusion of the antibody fragment to the pVIII capsid protein provides a multivalent display and can result in selection of phage through avidity rather than affinity[12] and stringent selection procedures must be used to identify high affinity binders.[13]

Phagemid vectors are replicated as single stranded DNA and then rescued as phage particles by co-infection with a helper phage.[14] Fewer copies of the antibody fusion product are displayed on the surface if phagemid/helper phage are used and this system provides a more stringent monovalent selection based on affinity.[15] The phagemid vector is much smaller than the genomic phage and hence cloning is easier and allows the generation of larger libraries. Phagemid vectors are, therefore, the preferred methodology.

In the Fab and Fd formats, one chain is fused to the phage coat protein and the other chain is expressed as a soluble protein which is secreted into the periplasm of *E. coli* where it links to the fused chain during assembly of phage particles.

Selection of Phage

Phage can be selected directly by antigen coupled to solid phases such as sepharose or plastic wells or against target cell surfaces or indirectly using soluble biotinylated antigen and subsequently captured by streptavidin coated beads. Methodologies for selection have been reviewed.[12-15] In addition, libraries can be pre-absorbed to remove non-target phage before the final antigen driven selection. This method is particularly useful in selecting phage which bind to the surface of specific cell types such as red blood cells.[16]

HUMAN ANTIBODY GENE LIBRARIES

Human monoclonal antibody genes can be rescued by phage display from hybridomas or, alternatively, antibody gene repertoires can be constructed directly from donors (Fig. 7.2). Antibodies rescued in this way from immunized donors will include VH and VL genes from B cells which have undergone in vivo somatic mutation to provide high affinity antibodies. Though it cannot be certain that the VH/VL combinations of an individual B cell have

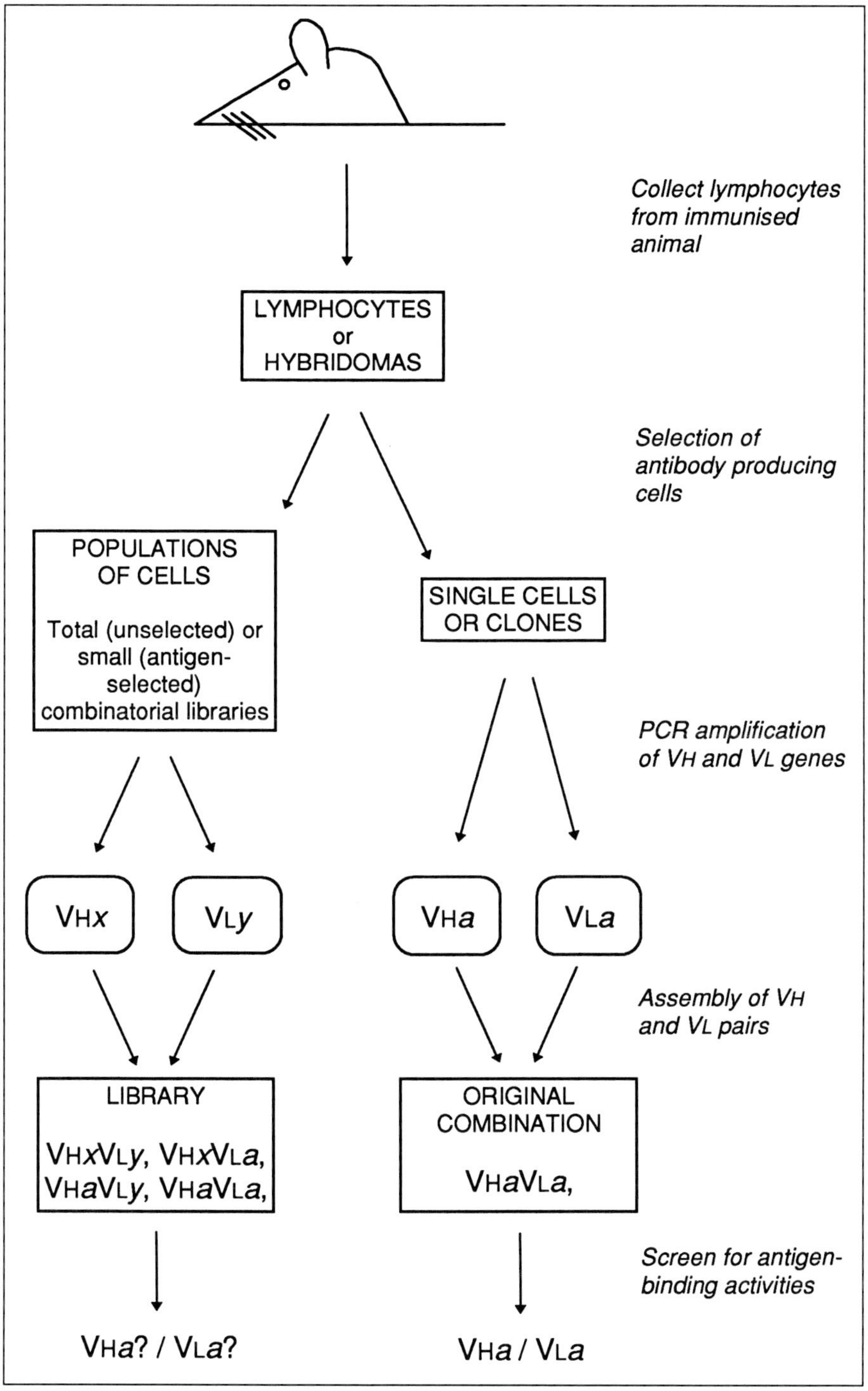

Fig. 7.2. Phage display of monoclonal antibody repertoire libraries. See text for details. Reproduced with permission from: Winter G, Milstein C. Man-made antibodies. Nature 1991; 349:293-299.

been reconstituted, this method has been successfully applied to isolate a range of human antibodies (Table 7.1). It is commonly found that a restricted number of between 1 and 3 different VH domain genes are isolated in association with between 4 to 7 different VL domain genes. Many antibodies of different specificity have been isolated from a library derived from the bone marrow of an individual.[17,18] For example, antibodies recognizing HIV, hepatitis B, RSV, CMV and herpes simplex type 1 were isolated from a long term asymptomatic HIV-1 patient.[17] Some of these antibodies have been shown to possess neutralizing activity (Table 7.1).

Mature human libraries from healthy individuals will not possess antibodies with affinities against self since they will have been deleted during maturation. Also, it is argued that libraries derived from adults will possess antigen binding sites which have undergone too much maturation and would need to be remodeled to bind new antigens.[1] To isolate human antibodies against new antigens, therefore, libraries described as naive have been constructed from unimmunized healthy donors[18] constructed semi-synthetically[19] or based upon germ line genes.[20] These have allowed the isolation of some antibodies against self antigens.[18,23] Antibodies selected from these naive libraries generally have association constants of 0.1-1.0 μM as expected from the primary immune response (Table 7.2).

Table 7.1. Human antibodies from immunized donors

Antigen	Biological activity	Reference
Hepatitis B	ND	37
HIV-I	+	30,38
Respiratory Syncytial Virus (RSV)	+	39,41
Cytomegalovirus	ND	17
Herpes simplex virus-I	+	17
Herpes simplex virus-2	+	17
Varicella zoster virus	ND	17
Measles	ND	17
Rubella	ND	17
Tetanus	ND	40
Thyroid peroxidase	ND	42

LARGE COMBINATORIAL LIBRARIES OF VH AND VL DOMAIN GENES

Human VH/VL genetic repertoires have the potential to generate 10^{10} possible combinations. This is far in excess of what is possible in a practical phage library which is limited to about 10^8 phage. As a way of increasing library size, Hoogenboom and colleagues[21] cloned the heavy and light chain repertoires on to separate replicon vectors, each being used to provide a library of 10^7. They were then brought together in *E. coli* to create the potential for up to 10^{14} VH/VL domain combinations. In order to package VH/VL domain combinations in the same phage particle the *cre/lox* site specific recombination system of coliphage P1 was used (Fig. 7.3). This has provided the basis for an excellent 'single pot' library of 10^{10} human VH/VL domain combinations[20] (Fig. 7.4) (see below).

SEMI-SYNTHETIC ANTIBODY LIBRARIES

A totally synthetic library could be constructed by replacing all six CDRs from a natural antibody with random sequences of amino acids. This complex task has not been undertaken to date and is likely to be unnecessary since a mouse can recognize an apparently unlimited number of antigens with a repertoire of 10^8 members.[22]

Two approaches have been taken to provide semi-synthetic libraries. Since CDR3-H and CDR3-L contribute most in terms of antigen binding (chapter 2), it has been argued that one could improve upon natural genetic diversity by chemically constructing random polypeptide combinations as CDR3s. Barbas and colleagues[19] started with a human antibody Fab fragment and replaced CDR3 H with random peptides. In one example, the anti-tetanus toxoid antibody 7E was displayed as an Fd fragment upon the

Table 7.2. Human antibodies from unimmunized donors

Antigen	Kd (M)	Reference
Thyroglobulin	4.3×10^{-6}	18
Red blood cells (fog-1)	9.3×10^{-6}	18
TNFα	6.4×10^{-6}	18
Carcinoembryonic antigen	ND	18
muc-1 (tumor mucins)	ND	18
CD4	ND	18

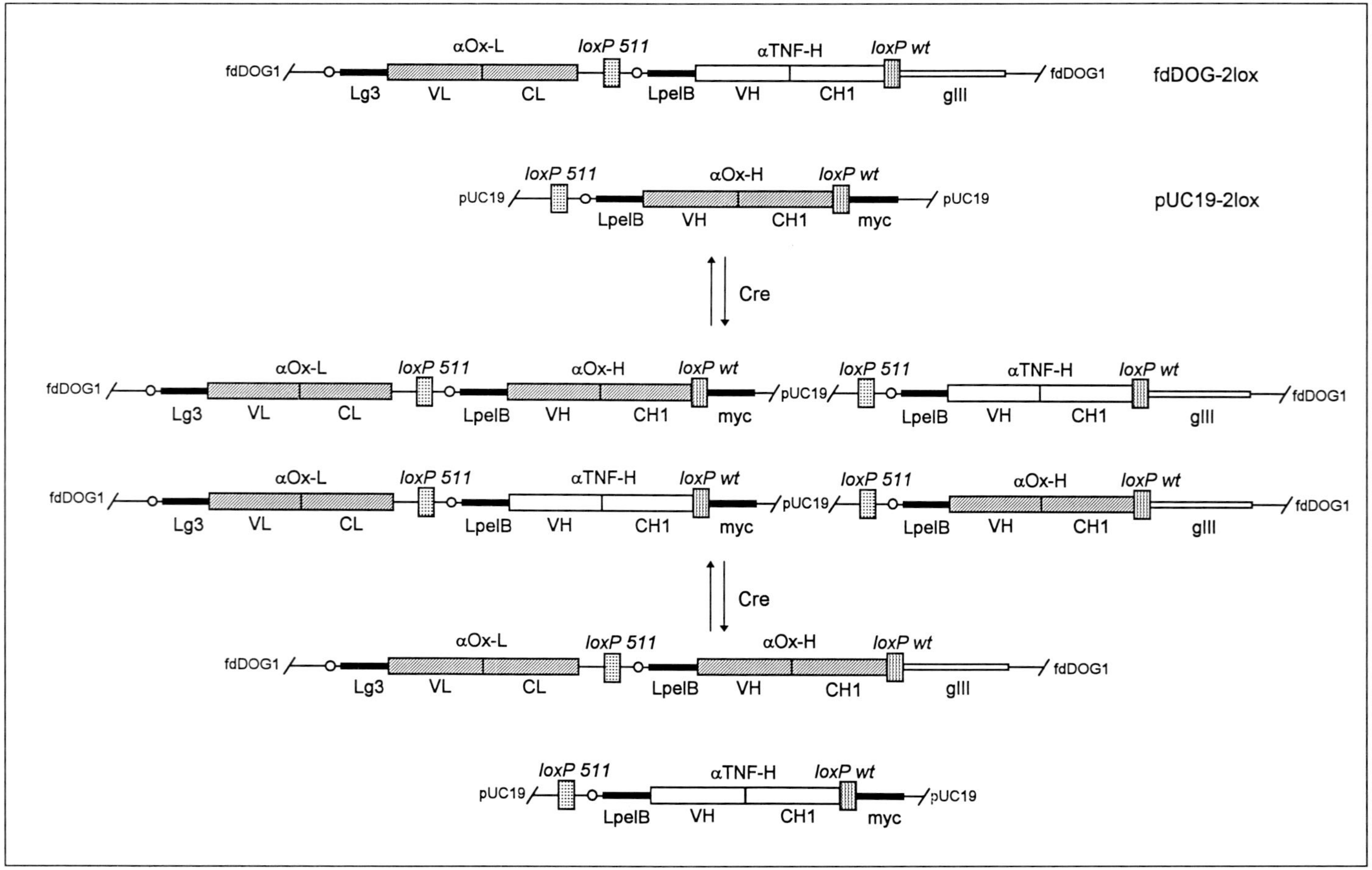

Fig. 7.3. The lox-Cre *site specific recombination system. In this simplified example, using defined domains rather than repertoires, replicons are generated by Cre mediated recombination between the acceptor phage vector fdDOG-2lox and the donor plasmid vector pUC19-2lox. fdDOG-2lox contains aVκ from a mouse anti-phOx antibody linked to a human Cκ constant domain and VH from the mouse anti-TNFα antibody mAb32 linked to a human Cμ constant domain. pUC19-2lox has VH of NQ10.12.5 linked to the human Cγ1 domain. Within* E. coli *an equilibrium between the six vectors develops due to the reversible nature of recombination in the* lox-Cre *system. Ribosome binding sites (o), c-myc peptide tag (myc), phage fd gene III leader sequence (Lg3),* pelB *leader sequence (LpelB), fd phage gene III (gIII), mutant* loxP 511 *and wild type* loxP wt *are indicated. The mutant* loxP 511 *prevents recombination within the same vector and subsequent loss of VH genes in the presence of Cre. Adapted from ref. 43.*

phagemid pComb3. PCR was used to replace the nucleotide sequence of the endogenous CDR3-H with the sequence $(NNS)_{16}$ i.e., 16 triplet repeats where N is A,C,G,T and S is G or C. This created a population of Fd fragments with CDR3-Hs of 16 randomly arranged amino acids, the other 5 CDRs of the parental anti-tetanus Fd being unchanged. The theoretical number of peptide sequences which could be generated is greater than 10^{20}. However, the maximum practical phage library size limited the diversity of CDR3-H to 5×10^{7}. Phage which bound fluorescein with Kd values of 0.1 μM were successfully selected. The original clone 7E which bound tetanus with a Kd of 0.1 μM had no affinity for fluorescein. Thus, replacing CDR3-H allowed the conversion from tetanus binding to fluorescein binding. The same parental antibody has also been used with synthetic CDR3-Hs to identify antibodies against integrins.[23]

A more diverse antibody library has been constructed by Griffiths et al[20] and is illustrated in Figure 7.4. The library is based upon the large combinatorial repertoire of human VH/VL domain combinations discussed above. The VH gene segment repertoire was combined with synthetic randomized CDR3-H loops of 4 to 12 residues, and the Vκ\λ gene segment repertoire combined with CDR3-L loops of 8-10 amino acid residues with 1, 2 or 3 random amino acid sequences. A Vκ\λ gene library was also constructed from 21 cloned Vκ\λ segments and a CDR3-L of 8 to 13 residues with 1 to 5 residues of random sequence. It is estimated that the resulting library has 6.5×10^{10} different phage combinations. This single pot library provided antibodies to 35 diverse antigens including haptens and protein antigens such as tubulin, gp120, calmodulin, human TNFα and thyroglobulin.[24] A list of antibodies identified against antigens of potential therapeutic interest is presented in Table 7.3.

AFFINITY IMPROVEMENT

Two approaches have been adopted to increase the affinity of antibodies displayed on phage.

MUTAGENESIS

In vivo affinity maturation can be mimicked in vitro by random mutagenesis within CDRs using error prone PCR[14,25,26] but this approach is severely limited by the number of mutants which

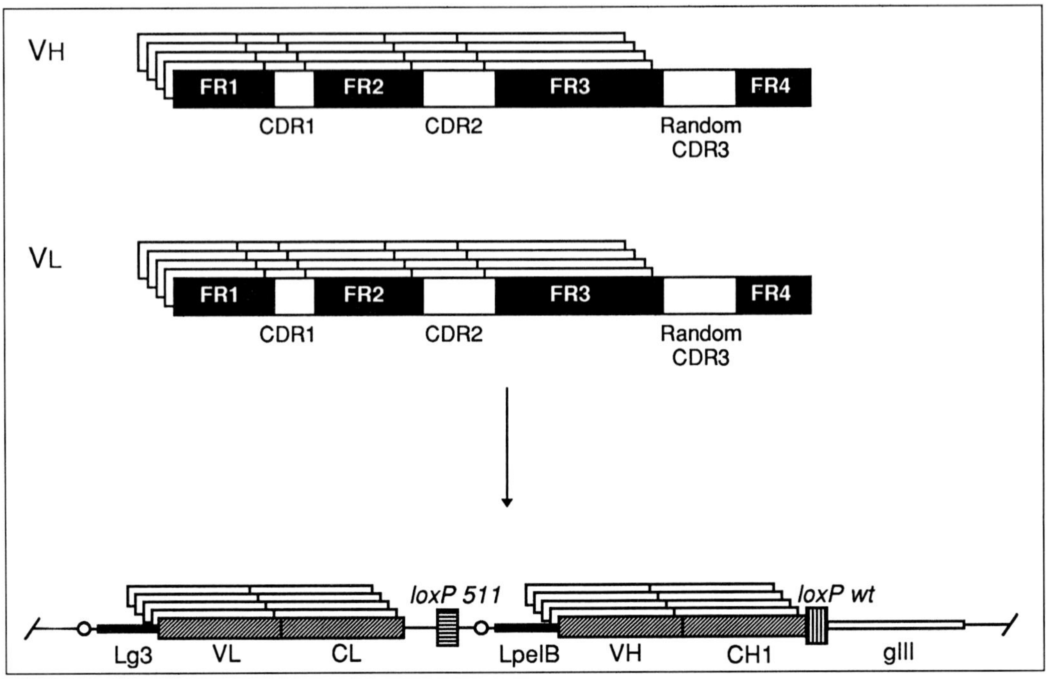

Fig. 7.4. Construction of semi-synthetic phage display libraries. See text for details. Reproduced with permission from: Griffiths AD, Williams SC, Hartlkey O et al. Isolation of high affinity human antibodies directly from large synthetic repertoires. EMBO J 1994; 13:3245-3260.

Table 7.3. Anti-human antibodies from synthetic libraries

Antigen	Reference
TNFα	20
Thyroglobulin	20
FcεR1	20
Tissue plasminogen activator	20
Urokinase	20
Plasmin	20
Carcinoembryonic antigen	20
c-erb-2	20
Factor VIII	20
Rhesus D	24
p53	24
SRY (human sex determining Y factor)	24
Anti-B	16
Anti-H1	16
Anti-rhesus D	16
Anti-E	16
Anti-Kp	16
Ery.X1 (panagglutinin)	16
Integrins	23

can be screened. A computer assisted method of pre-selecting mutated sites has been described[27] but even then, randomization of just six codons provides the 10^9 combinations to saturate a standard phage library size.[28] Mutagenesis by growth in mutator strains of *E. coli* has also been suggested though not undertaken to date.

Chain Shuffling

The early work which analyzed diversity within phage display libraries clearly showed promiscuity with respect to functional VH-VL combinations and in particular a single VH could pair with several VL chains and still retain antigen binding.[29,30] Chain shuffling has therefore been used to generate new combinations.[31] In one laboratory example, a human phage antibody against 2-phenyl oxazolone-5-one (phOX) with an affinity of 3.2×10^{-7} M, was isolated from a library derived from an unimmunized donor. Shuffling the light chains increased affinity 20-fold and shuffling the heavy chains increased affinity by a further 15-fold.[32]

EPITOPE IMPRINTING

As discussed previously (chapter 6), rodent antibody repertoires provide a rich source of high affinity monoclonals and humanization of these is providing a rich new supply of therapeutics. An alternate way of isolating a human equivalent of a rodent monoclonal antibody using the phage display technique has been described and is known as epitope imprinting.[6] This is illustrated in Figure 7.5. The method is an extension of the chain shuffling technique whereby a rodent monoclonal antibody of potential therapeutic interest is displayed on a phage and then the heavy and light antibody chains from human VH and VL libraries are sequentially shuffled upon the phage. Selection by panning with antigen at each stage ensures isolation of phage which retain binding affinity for the same antigen as the original rodent monoclonal. The method relies on efficient pairing between rodent VH and human VL and vice versa. Since these association constants are in the range of 10^{4-6} M^{-1}, the antibody is displayed in the Fab format so that additional association can be provided by CH1 and CL domains. Using this technique, Jespers and colleagues[33] isolated a human Fab fragment against TNFα which had an affinity Kd of 15 nM compared with 26 nM binding of the rodent antibody originally displayed on the phage.

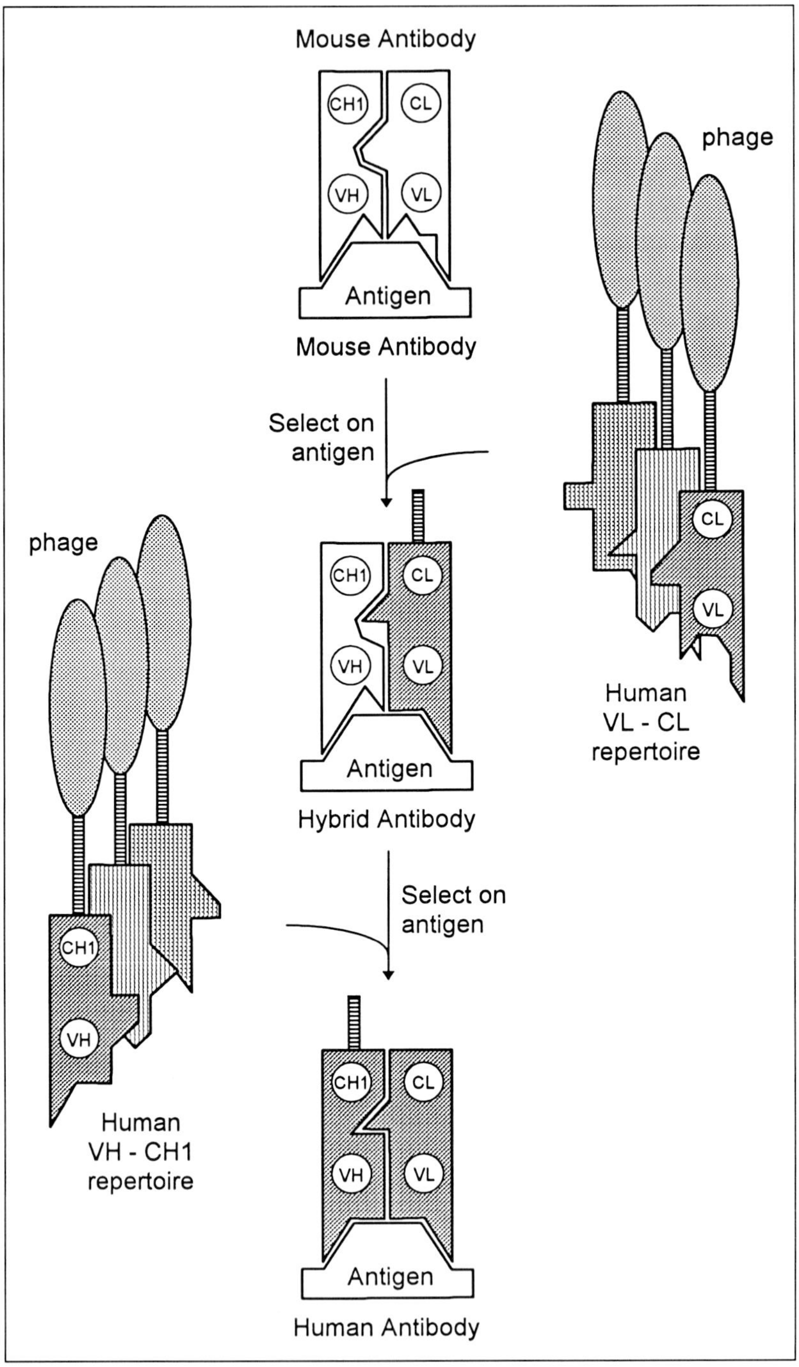

Fig. 7.5. Epitope imprinting to select a human antibody recognizing the same epitope as a murine antibody. The progenitor mouse antibody is displayed on the surface of phage in an Fab format. The murine VL is first replaced by chain shuffling with a human VL library and then the murine VH replaced by chain shuffling with a human VH library. Adapted with permission from: Jespers LS, Roberts A, Mahler SM et al. Guiding the selection of human antibodies from a phage display repertoire to a single epitope of an antigen. Biotechnology 1994; 12:899-903.

THE FUTURE OF THERAPEUTICS FROM PHAGE DISPLAY LIBRARIES

Since the first description of the technique of antibody display on phage in 1989 there has been a continual stream of scientific publications on both extending the scope of the technology and identifying phage which bind to a plethora of target antigens. The technology is also perceived as of significant commercial value and this has led to over-speculation that the technique can now completely replace the provision of monoclonal antibodies by other means.[34,35] The technology is, clearly, a very powerful method of identifying antibody-based antigen binding domains against virtually any target antigen that is available for affinity purification of the phage.

Some caution should be taken, however, in the pursuit of human therapeutics particularly with respect to the nature of the combinatorial library and the method used to identify high affinity antibodies, bearing in mind that therapeutics should be immuno-silent. We are still uncertain as to the importance of the relative orientation of antigen-antibody interactions and biological activity.

The most expedient approach is the recovery of high affinity antibodies from a library derived from an individual immunized with the target antigen, but this approach is limited by the scope of immunization possible. The use of a naive library derived from unimmunized individuals should provide immunosilent antibodies, but this library is likely to yield only low affinity antibodies. Chain shuffling within such a library may increase affinity but this has not been reproducibly demonstrated. The alternative approach of in vitro mutagenesis is likely to increase affinity though it equally raises the opportunity for the introduction of immunogenic epitopes.

The semi-synthetic libraries derive much of their diversity from the synthetic CDR3-H and CDR3-L. It can be argued that since in vivo CDR3s are derived by recombination, synthetic CDRs are merely a copy of this process. The latter CDRs have not, however, been exposed in vivo to self/non-self discrimination. High affinity antibodies selected from semi-synthetic libraries are likely to attribute most of their binding affinity to interaction through the synthetic CDR3s in contrast to natural high affinity antibodies which use on average four to five CDRs (see chapter 2). The biological significance of this different orientation of antigen-antibody interaction is unknown. A seminal example is described by Kelley and colleagues[36] who prepared humanized variants of the p185-her antibody which recognizes breast and ovarian tumors. They described a humanized variant which had the same binding affinity as the chimeric antibody but very different enthalpy changes on binding to antigen. The chimeric antibody had anti-proliferative activity but the humanized variant did not. Selection based upon affinity may therefore yield antibodies which are not therapeutically effective.

Despite these qualifications, one can look forward to a series of therapeutics derived from phage libraries. The technology is in its infancy and therapeutics are several years from the clinic. It would not be surprising, however, if the first of such products were antibodies derived from immunized donors.

References

1. Winter G, Milstein C. Man-made antibodies. Nature 1991; 349:293-299.
2. Betz AG, Neuberger MS, Milstein,C. Discriminating intrinsic and antigen-selected mutational hotspots in immunoglobulin V genes. Immunology Today. 1993; 14:405-411.
3. Huse WD, Sastry L, Iverson SA et al. Generation of a large combinatorial library of immunoglobulin repertoire in phage lambda. Science 1989; 246:1275-1281.
4. Gussow D, Ward ES, Griffiths PT et al. Generating binding activities from *E. coli* by expression of a repertoire of immunoglobulin variable domains. Cold Spring Harbour Symp Quant Biol 1989; LIV:265-271.
5. Chang CN, Landolfi NF, Queen C. Expression of antibody Fab domains on bacteriophage surfaces. J Immunol 1991; 147: 3610-3614.
6. Winter G, Griffiths AD, Hawkins RE et al. Making antibodies by phage display technology. Ann Rev Immunol 1994; 12:433-455.
7. Huse WD. In: Borrebaeck, CAK, ed. Antibody Engineering. A Practical Guide. New York: WH Freeman & Co, 1992:103-120.
8. Hoogenboom HR, Marks JD, Griffiths AD et al. Building antibodies from their genes. Immunol Rev 1992; 130:41-68.
9. McCafferty J, Griffiths AD, Winter G et al. Phage antibodies: filamentous phage displaying antibody variable domains. Nature 1990; 348:552-554.
10. Barbas CF, Kang AS, Lerner RA et al. Assembly of combinatorial antibody libraries on phage surfaces: the gene III site. Proc Nat Acad Sci 1991; 8:7978-7982.

11. Huse WD, Stinchcombe TJ, Glaser SM et al. Appication of a filamentous phage pVIII fusion protein system suitable for efficient production, screening and mutagenesis of Fab antibody fragments. J Biol Chem 1992; 149:3914-3920.
12. Smith GP. Surface presentation of protein epitopes using bacteriophage systems. Curr Opin Biotechnol 1991; 2:668-673.
13. Barrett RW, Cwirla SE, Ackerman MS et al. Selective enrichment and characterisation of high affinity ligands from collections of random peptides on filamentous phage. Anal Biochem 1992; 204:357-364.
14. Soderlind E, Simonsson AC, Borrebaeck CAK. Phage display technology in antibody engineering: design of phagemid vetors and *in vitro* maturation systems. Immunol Rev 1992; 130:109-124.
15. Garrard LJ, Yang M, O'Conell MP et al. Fab assembly and enrichment in a monovalent phage display system. Biotechnology 1991; 9:1373-1372.
16. Marks JD, Ouwehand WH, Bye JM et al. Human antibody fragments specific for human blood group antigens from a phage display library. Biotechnology 1993; 1:1145-1149.
17. Williamson RA, Burioni R, Sanna PP et al. Human monoclonal antibodies against a plethora of viral pathogens from single combinatorial libraries. Proc Nat Acad Sci 1993; 90:4141-4145.
18. Griffiths AD, Malmquist M, Marksa JD et al. Human anti-self antibodies with high specificity from phage display libraries. EMBO J 1993; 12:725-734.
19. Barbas CF, Bain JD, Hoekstra DM et al. Semisynthetic combinatorial libraries: a chemical solution to the diversity problem. Proc Nat Acad Sci 1992; 89:4457-4461.
20. Griffiths AD, Williams SC, Hartlkey O et al. Isolation of high affinity human antibodies directly from large synthetic repertoires. EMBO J 1994; 13:3245-3260.
21. Hoogenboom HR, Griffiths AD, Johnson WKS et al. Multi-subunit proteins on the surface of filamentous phage: methodologies for displaying antibody (Fab) heavy and light chains. Nucl Acid Res 1991; 19:4133-4137.
22. Berek C, Milstein C. Mutation drift and repertoire shift in the maturation of the immune response. Immunol Rev 1987; 10:5-26.
23. Barbas CF, Languino LR, Smith JW. High affinity self-reactive human antibodies by design and selection: targeting the integrin ligand binding site. Proc Nat Acad Sci 1993; 90:10003-10007.
24. Nissim A, Hoogenbum HR, Tomlinson IM et al. Antibody fragments from a single pot phage display library as immunochemical reagents. EMBO J 1994; 13:692-698.
25. Glaser SM, Yelton DE, Huse WD. Antibody engineering by codon-based mutagenesis in a filamentous phage vector system. J Immunol 1992; 149:3903-3913.

26. Hawkins RE, Russell SJ, Winter G. Selection of phage antibodies by binding affinity: mimicking affinity maturation. J Mol Biol 1992; 226:889-896.
27. Balint RF, Larrick JW. Antibody engineering by parsimonious mutagenesis. Gene 1993; 137:109-118.
28. Clackson T, James A. *In vitro* selection from protein and peptide libraries. Trends Biotech 1994; 12:173-184.
29. Clackson T, Hoogenboom HR, Griffiths AD et al. Making antibody fragments using phage display libraries. Nature 1991; 352:624-628.
30. Burton DR, Barbas CF, Persson MAA et al. A large array of human monoclonal antibodies to type 1 human immunodeficiency virus from combinatorial libraries of asymptomatic individuals. Proc Nat Acad Sci 1991; 88:10134-10137.
31. Kang AS, Jones TM, Burton DR. Antibody redesign by chain shuffling from random combinatorial libraries. Proc Nat Acad Sci 1991; 88:11120-11123.
32. Marks JD, Griffiths AD, Malmquist M et al. By-passing immunisation: building high affinity human antibodies by chain shuffling. Biotechnology 1992; 10:779-783.
33. Jespers LS, Roberts A, Mahler SM et al. Guiding the selection of human antibodies from a phage display repertoire to a single epitope of an antigen. Biotechnology 1994; 12:899-903.
34. Chiswell DJ, McCafferty J. Phage antibodies: will new "coliclonal" antibodies replace monoclonal antibodies? Trends Biotech 1992; 10:80-84.
35. Lerner RA, Kang AS, Bain JD et al. Antibodies without immunisation. Science 1992; 258:1313-1314.
36. Kelley RF, O'Connell MP, Carter P et al. Antigen binding thermodynamics and anti-proliferative effects of chimeric and humanised anti-p185-her2 antibody Fab fragments. Biochemistry 1992; 31:5434-5441.
37. Zebedee SL, Barbas CF, Hom Y-L et al. Human combinatorial antibody libraries to hepatitis B surface antigen. Proc Nat Acad Sci 1992; 89:3175-3179.
38. Barbas CF, Bjorling E, Chiodi F et al. Recombinant human Fab fragments neutralise human type 1 immunodeficiency virus *in vitro*. Proc Nat Acad Sci 1992; 89:9339-9343.
39. Barbas CF, Crowe JR, Cababa D et al. Human monoclonal Fab fragments derived from a combinatorial library bind to respiratory syncytial virus F glycoprotein and neutralise infectivity. Proc Nat Acad Sci 1992; 89:10164-10168.
40. Mullinax RL, Gross EA, Amberg JR et al. Identification of human antibody fragment clones specific for tetanus toxoid in a bacteriophage lambda immunoexpression library. Proc Nat Acad Sci 1990; 87:8095-8099.

41. Crowe JE, Murphy BR, Chanock RM et al. Recombinant human respiratory syncytial virus monoclonal antibody Fab is effective therapeutically when introduced directly into the lungs of RSV-infected mice. Proc Nat Acad Sci 1994; 91:1386-1390
42. Portolano S, McLachlan SM, Rapoport B. High affinity, thyroid specific human autoantibodies displayed on the surface of filamentous phage use V genes similar to other autoantibodies. J Immunol 1993; 151:2839-2851.
43. Waterhouse P, Griffiths AD, Johnson K et al. Combinatorial infection and *in vivo* recombination: a strategy for making large phage antibody repertoires. Nuc Acid Res 1993; 21:2265-2266.

CHAPTER 8

Transgenic Mice with Human Immunoglobulins

INTRODUCTION

Transgenic animals are defined as animals that carry foreign genes integrated within the chromosomes of their germ line. While all the cells of the animal carry the genetic information of the foreign gene, selective tissue specific expression can be achieved by incorporating genetic signals from the host animal for tissue specific promoters and enhancers adjacent to the structural gene of the foreign protein. The advent of transgenic mouse technology has had a major impact upon medical research and offers new ways of identifying and evaluating human therapeutics.[1] Technology is now being adopted to create transgenic mice carrying human immunoglobulin genes in germline configurations.

The entire repertoire of human heavy and kappa light chain genes are carried upon a 2.5 mega-base segment of chromosome 14 and a 2.0 mega-base component of chromosome 2 respectively. It is a major challenge to introduce such large segments of DNA into the mouse genome. This has not been achieved to date. A promising beginning has, however, been made. Early studies used artificially constructed plasmids or cosmids carrying some immunoglobulin heavy chains which were microinjected into mouse embryos (Fig. 8.1) and this created mice that expressed human

Antibody Therapeutics, by William J. Harris and Charles Cunningham. © 1995 R.G. Landes Company.

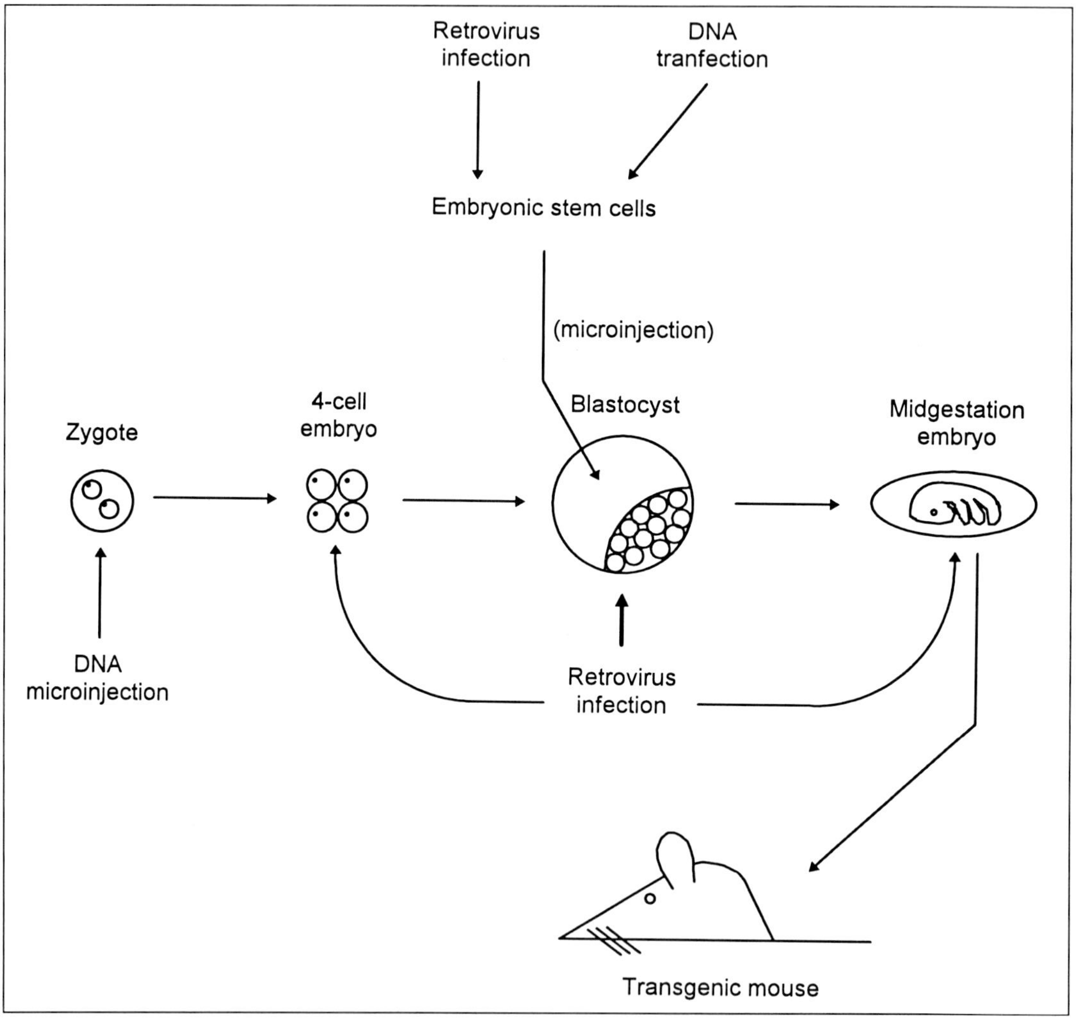

Fig. 8.1. Methods of generating transgenic mice. DNA can be microinjected into zygotes or introduced into embryonic stem cells, early developing embryos or blastocysts using retroviral vectors. Adapted with permission from: Gridley T, Soriano P Jaenisch R et al. Insertional mutagenesis in mice. Trends in Genetics 1989; 3:162-166; © Elsevier Trends Journals, Cambridge.

immunoglobulin heavy chains.[2-5] Larger mini-loci have been similarly constructed in yeast artificial chromosomes (YACs)[6,7] and this has allowed the expression of mini-loci carrying either a few heavy chain or light chain genes in transgenic mice. These mini-loci undergo lymphoid specific gene rearrangements and the transgenic mice develop B cells expressing human immunoglobulin polypeptide chains. If the mini-loci are introduced into mice which retain their capacity to make mouse immunoglobulins, the serum titers of human immunoglobulin are very low, usually below 1 mg/ml. It has been necessary therefore to eliminate the ability of the recipient mice to make mouse immunoglobulin through disruption of the endogenous immunogobulin loci.

The overall route to generating transgenic mice that make human immunoglobulins is depicted in Figure 8.2. Two mouse strains are developed in which the heavy or light chain genes are disabled by gene targeting. In addition, two transgenic mouse strains are made by introducing mini-loci carrying a few human heavy or light chain genes into recipient mice. All four mouse types are then cross bred until a unique mouse making only human immunoglobulin is derived. Two such strains have been developed commercially; one described as the 'HuMAB-Mouse' (GenPharm Inc.) and the other as the 'Xenomouse' (Cell Genesys Inc.).

DEVELOPMENT OF MICE DEFICIENT IN B CELLS

Targeted disruption of endogenous heavy and light chain genetic loci is achieved by introducing foreign genes into the loci thereby disrupting their overall structure. This is most easily done by transfecting a vector carrying a selectable marker into embryonic stem cells (ES cells; Fig. 8.1). One specific example of this is shown in Figure 8.3.[8] A vector carrying a neomycin resistance gene was electroporated into ES cells and those cells which incorporated the vector selected through their neomycin resistance. In this example, the neomycin resistant gene had replaced Jκ segments resulting in a mouse strain, JCKD, which cannot undergo VJ rearrangement and cannot, therefore, give rise to mature B cells.[8] A heavy chain mutant mouse JHD, in which the JH gene segments are deleted was similarly derived.[9] These two defective mutants have been used to derive the 'HuMAB mouse'.

Other defective mouse strains include the 'μMT' mutation in which the Cμ membrane exon is destroyed. Homozygous μMT/

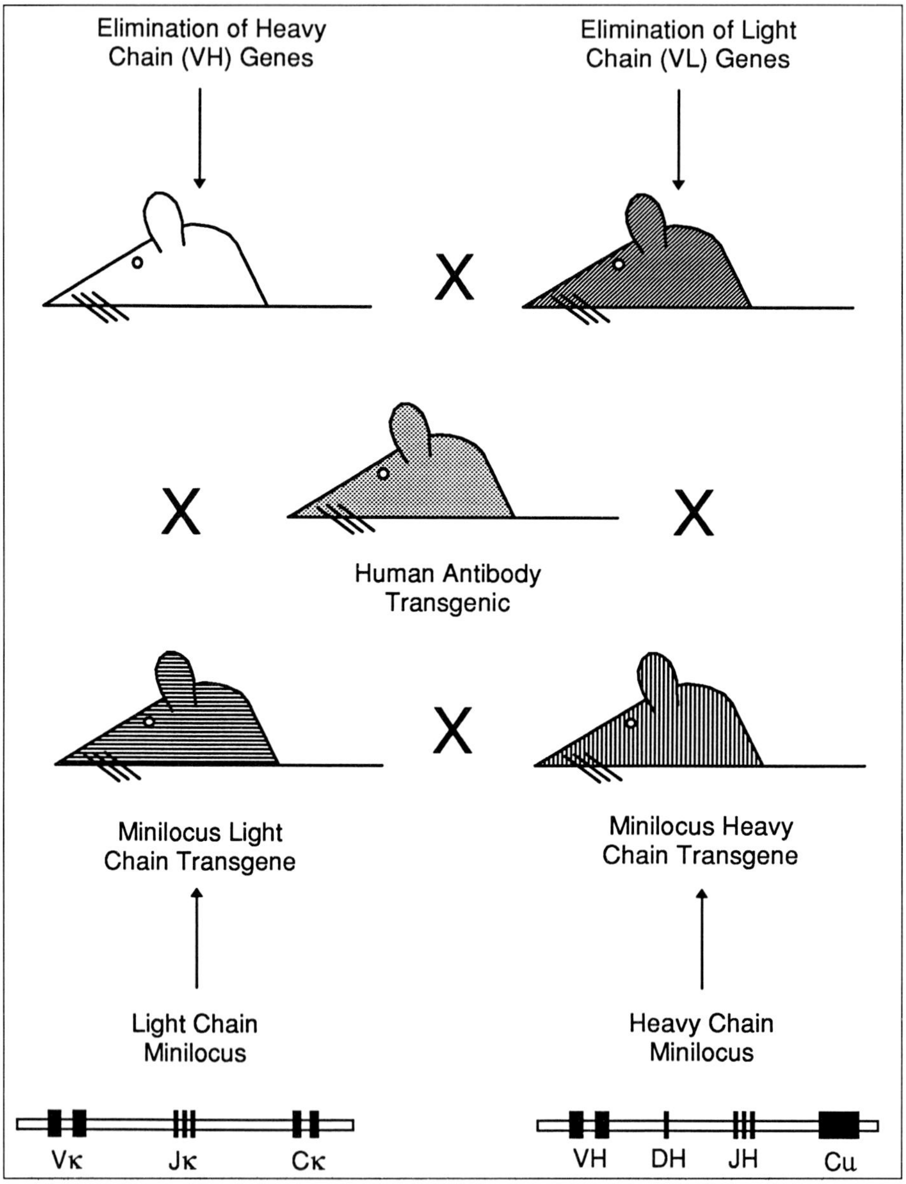

Fig. 8.2. Development of a transgenic mouse making only human immunoglobulin. Four different mice are generated. Knockout mice which cannot express VH or Vκ are made and two other strains are developed containing human VH and Vκ miniloci. A transgenic mouse expressing only human immunoglobulin can then be derived by sequential crossing and selection.

μMT mice cannot make the membrane form of Cμ which is essential for B cell development. Thus, these mice have no B cells or circulating antibody.[10]

MINI-LOCUS TRANSGENE CONSTRUCTS AND THEIR DIVERSITY

In order to assemble a human antibody chain, mini-loci must include VH, D and JH exons, a constant region gene and enhancer expression signals for VH assembly and Vκ\λ, Jκ\λ and Cκ\λ regions for light chain expression. The breadth of the repertoire of heavy and light chains which can be assembled is determined by the gene diversity within the mini-loci. Figure 8.4 lists the mini-loci which have been introduced into transgenics and these are discussed in more detail below.

HuIgH and HuIgH cos

The HuIgH mini-locus, which contains two VH gene segments (VH26 and VH186), one human D segment and three synthetic

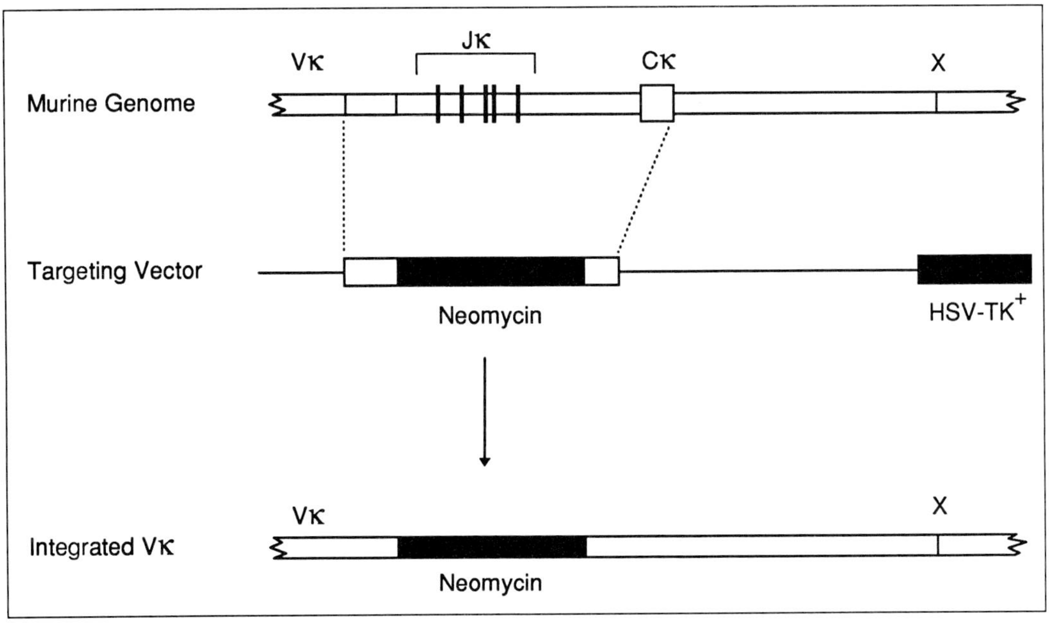

Fig. 8.3. Generation of a knockout mouse deficient in synthesis of murine Vκ. A gene vector is constructed containing a part of the Vκ locus disrupted by the insertion of the gene for neomcyin resistance. This vector is introduced into ES cells and those inheriting the vector selected by drug resistance. Resulting mice are then screened for lack of expression of Vκ chains. Adapted from: Chen J, Trounstine M, Kurahara C et al. B cell development in mice that lack one or both immunoglobulin K light chain genes. EMBO J 1993; 12:821-830.

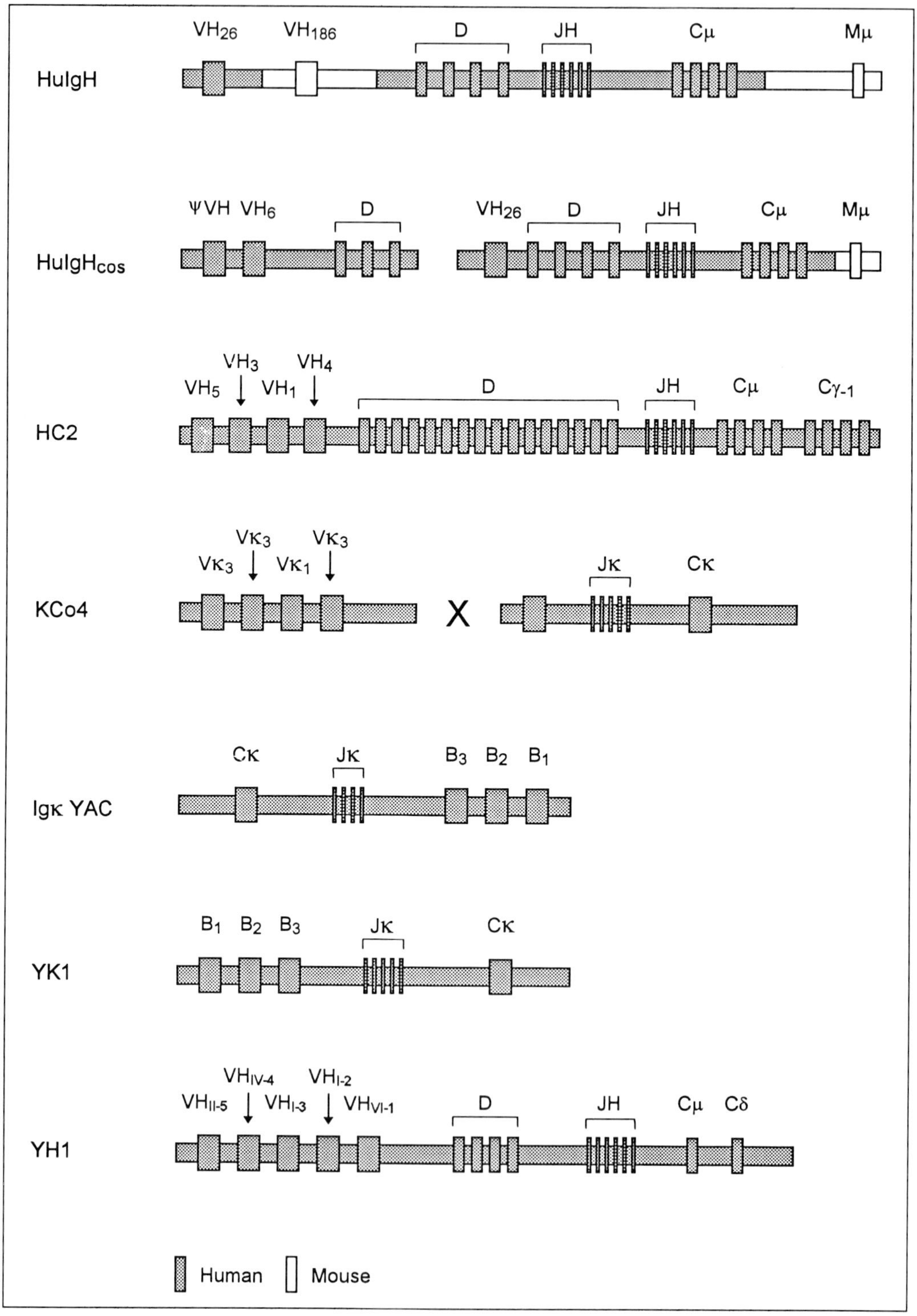

Fig. 8.4. Representative examples of miniloci which have been introduced into transgenic mice. See text for details.

D segments, six JH segments as well as the Cμ locus[2] were introduced into the μMT mouse and homozygotes selected by intercrossing the F_1 generation. Resulting transgenics incorporated 3-5 copies of the mini-locus into the genome and had on the order of 100-450 μg/ml of HuIgM heavy chains in their sera.[11]

Equivalent levels of human IgM are found in homozygous transgenics possessing HuIgHcos which includes seven D segments in addition to ψVH, VH6, VH26 and six JH segments.[3] Sequence analysis of the VH26 rearranged genes present in spleen cells showed about 70% of the rearrangements to contain frameshifts or stop codons which would not give rise to protein. This is likely to arise through multiple copies of HuIgHcos being present in the genome. Nevertheless, rearrangements based upon the use of multiple segments and diversity at V-D-J junctions confirmed assembly and expression of diverse human heavy chains.[11]

HC2

The HC2 mini-locus consists of an 80 kilobase DNA fragment containing four human V germ line segments (VH1(51p1), VH3(56p1), VH4(4.21), VH5(25.1)), 15 D segments, six JH segments, Cμ and Cγ1 as well as enhancer and switch regions.[12] Transgenic mice containing this mini-locus have both human IgM and IgG_1 heavy chains in their serum and it has been shown that the IgG_1 arises through authentic class switching.

KCo4

KCo4 consists of two mini-loci which share a common 3 kb sequence. When the two plasmids were co-injected, homologous recombination occurred and the two mini-loci integrated as a contiguous 43 kb segment comprising four V segments (Vκ1 and Vκ3, 65.3, 65.5 and 65.8), five Jκ segments, the Cκ exon and enhancer elements.[13]

IGκ YAC

The ability of YACs to contain very large segments of DNA has been exploited to isolate a YAC which contains a 300 kb insert of the human κ immunoglobulin locus from a human library.[7] This insert includes 3 Vκ segments, the intact Jκ cluster, the Cκ region and enhancer. The YAC was modified to include selectable markers and introduced into murine ES cells by protoplast fusion.

The ES cells were then injected into blastocysts. A chimeric mouse was identified in which 40% of its cells contained the Igκ YAC. A titer of 3 mg/ml of human κ chain was found in the serum. These included a mixture of V-J rearrangements.

YH1/YK1

yH1 is a YAC containing a 220 kb segment of the human immunoglobulin VH locus and includes five VH genes (VH_{II-5}, VH_{IV-4}, VH_{I-3}, VH_{I-2} and VH_{VI-1}), four D segments, the six functional JH regions, Cμ and Cδ regions and an enhancer. yK1 contains a 170 kb segment of the human immunoglobulin κ locus and includes three Vκ genes from the B cluster (B1, B2 and B3), all five functional Jκ regions, the Cκ region, enhancers and the κ deleting element. These were separately introduced into murine ES cells by protoplast fusion and YAC-containing chimeric mice generated.[14] Offspring containing yH1 and yK1 in their germ lines were then identified and found to have serum levels only of the order of 0.4 - 1.0 mg/ml of human μ chain and 10-30 mg/ml of human κ chains when the recipient mice still retained intact endogenous immunoglobulin loci. Serum levels of 350 mg/ml of human μ chains were, however, obtained when transgenes were constructed in mice deficient in mouse heavy chain development (yH-1; JH/JH).[4]

TRANSGENIC MICE MAKING INTACT HUMAN ANTIBODIES

Transgenic mice possessing the HC2 and KCo4 mini-loci have been cross-bred with mutant strains JHD and JCKD and double transgenic/double deletion mutant mice derived.[13] Human IgM expressing cells are found in the spleen, lymph nodes, peritoneum and bone marrow of these animals although the absolute number of B cells in bone marrow and spleen is 10-50% lower than normal. Serum levels of the order of 100 mg/ml human μ heavy chain and κ light chain and 1 mg/ml of human γ heavy chain were observed. Furthermore, analysis of the VH sequences of IgG secreting clones has shown about 2% to include non-germline encoded sequences. Thus, class switching and somatic mutation of human genes both occur in these transgenic mice. Although the transgenes carry four different human VH genes, there was strong preferential usage of the VH3 family gene and no apparent use of VH5.

These mice, however, also produce murine heavy and light antibody chains at serum levels of the order of 1-10 mg/ml. Elimination of this endogenous chain production will require more extensive deletion of the murine immunoglobulin loci.

Antigen specific human IgM, then human IgG, arose after immunization with either human IgE or human CD4 as expected in a normal immune response.[13] Hybridomas derived from the spleen of these immunized animals produced human IgG monoclonal antibodies with affinities of the order of 9×10^{-7} M.

Transgenic mice (yH1:yK1) have also been generated by mating yH1 and yK1 bearing mice.[14] These mice produced a range of human VH and Vκ chains which made use of all D, JH and Jκ segments included in the YACs from which they were derived. Three of the four VH genes were used, with a much higher usage of V1v. V11, which is located close to the YAC cloning site, was not used. All three Vκ genes were used but there was a very strong bias towards one (B3) which was represented in about 80% of all Vκ composite genes. Only 50% of Vκ genes were in frame and could yield functional polypeptide chains. N additions at both V-D and D-J junctions were observed and the majority of in-frame clones contained a CDR3 of 10-18 amino acids in VH, and 9-10 amino acids in Vκ, as expected from normal B cell development.

yH1:yK1 transgenic mice have been immunized with tetanus toxoid C fragment (tetC) and tetC-specific antibodies detected in the sera. These transgenes have been developed in immunoglobulin-competent mice, hence their sera contains antibodies derived from murine and human heavy and light chains. Only 4% of hybridomas derived from immunized mice secreted entirely human anti-tetC monoclonal antibodies.

yH-1:yK-1(JH/JH; Cκ/Cκ) transgenic mice ('Xenomouse') contain two functionally inactivated mouse heavy and κ light chain alleles and produce entirely human antibodies (Hμ/Hκ) or antibodies made up from the human heavy chain and mouse λ light chains. Serum levels up to 200 mg/ml of Hμ/Hκ antibodies have been found in some Xenomouse strains.[14]

DIVERSITY OF USAGE OF V GENES

An important factor in determining the range of human antibodies which may possibly be derived from transgenic mice is the level of structural diversity achievable through the availability of only two to four VH genes. Studies to date have demonstrated diversity through junctional and combinatorial processes with a selection of D and JH genes, and somatic mutation has been observed. The pattern of VH, D and JH segment usage in YAC containing transgenic mice[14] more closely mirrored adult human B cell development than immunoglobulin mini-gene bearing mice[3-5] which showed position-biased VH and D usage. Furthermore, the average length of N addition (6.1 bp) within YAC-bearing mice closely approximates that found in adult human B cells (7.7 bp) while the average length of 2.9 bp in mini-loci bearing mice resembles that seen in adult mouse B cells.[14] This suggests that elements within the larger human genomic fragments in YACs carry nucleotide sequences to direct human-like combinatorial assembly of immunoglobulins.

The natural human VH and Vκ loci include about 46 functional VH and 35 functional Vκ germ line genes and the introduction of this extensive repertoire into a transgenic mouse is unlikely in the near future. The human germline repertoire is limited to seven sub-families, though nearly 50% belong to the VH3 subfamily, and it has been suggested that the introduction of one member of each family along with junctional diversity and somatic hypermutation may be sufficient to provide an extensive repertoire.[11] However, the occurrence of significant hypermutation in these transgenics has not been demonstrated. Also, a low number of VH genes may result in low frequencies of productive rearrangements and incomplete B cell maturation, limiting the potential B cell repertoire.[15]

CONCLUSIONS

There has been significant progress in developing transgenic mice which possess B cells expressing antibodies derived entirely from human genetic information. It has been shown that immunization of these transgenic mice does result in the specific development of both IgM and IgG antibodies against the immunogen and that these antibodies can be of relatively high affinity. Only a small proportion of the human immunoglobulin complex has been incorporated into transgenic mice to date and only a few antigen specific monoclonal antibodies derived from them. It is unclear whether currently available transgenic mice offer an opportunity for therapeutic antibodies. The major role for transgenic mice is the provision of antibodies which will not be immunogenic in man.

Although combinatorial assembly and somatic mutation have been observed and closely resemble normal human immunoglobulin development, the assembly of human immunoglobulins is occurring against a background of in vivo self/non-self discrimination by the mouse. The immunosilence of such antibodies remains to be determined.

REFERENCES

1. Palmiter RD, Brinster RL. Germ-line transformation of mice. Ann Rev Genetics 1986; 20:465-499.
2. Bruggemann M, Caskey HM, Teale C et al. A repertoire of monoclonal antibodies with human heavy chains from transgenic mice. Proc Nat Acad Sci 1989; 86:6709-6713.
3. Bruggemann M, Spicer C, Buluwela L et al. Human antibody production in transgenic mice: expression from 100 kb of the human IgH locus. Eur J Immunol 1991; 21:1323-1326.
4. Tuaillon N, Taylor LD, Lonberg N et al. Human immunoglobulin heavy chain minilocus recombination in transgenic mice: gene segment use in μ and γ transcripts. Proc Nat Acad Sci 1993; 90:3720-3724.
5. Taylor LD, Carmack CE, Schramm SR et al. A transgenic mouse that expresses a diversity of human sequence heavy and light chain immunoglobulins. Nucleic Acid Res 1992; 20:6287-6295
6. Choi TK, Hollenbach PW, Pearson BE et al. Transgenic mice containing a human heavy chain immunoglobulin gene fragment cloned in a yeast artificial chromosome. Nature (Genetics) 1993; 4:117-123.
7. Davies NR, Rosewell IR, Richardson JR et al. Creation of mice expressing human antibody light chain by introduction of a yeast artifical chromosome containing the core region of the human immunoglobulin κ locus. Biotechnology 1993; 11:911-914.
8. Chen J, Trounstine M, Kurahara C et al. B cell development in mice that lack one or both immunoglobulin K light chain genes. EMBO J 1993; 12:821-830.
9. Chen J, Trounstine M, Alt FW et al. Immunoglobulin gene rearrangements in B cell deficient mice generated by targeted deletion of the JH locus. Int Immmunl 1993; 5:647-656.
10. Kitamura D, Roes J, Kuhn R et al. A B-cell deficient mouse by targeted disruption of the membrane exon of the immunoglobulin μ chain gene. Nature 1991; 350:423-426.
11. Wagner SD, Williams GT, Larson T et al. Antibodies generated from human immunoglobulin miniloci in transgenic mice. Nucleic Acids Res 1994; 22:1389-1393.
12. Taylor LD, Carmack CE, Huazar D et al. Human immunoglobulin transgenes undergo rearrangement, somatic mutation and class switching in mice that lack endogenous IgM. Int Immunol 1994; 6:579-591.

13. Lonberg N, Taylor LD, Harding FA et al. Antigen specific human antibodies from mice comprising four distinct genetic modifications. Nature 1994; 368:856-859.
14. Green LL, Hardy MC, Maynard-Currie CE et al. Antigen-specific human monoclonal antibodies from mice engineered with human Ig heavy and light chain YAC's. Nature (Genetics) 1994; 7:13-21.
15. Jakobovits A, Vergera GJ, Kennedy JL et al. Analysis of homozygous mutant chimeric mice: deletion of the immunoglobulin heavy chain joining region blocks B cell development and antibody production. Proc Nat Acad Sci 1993; 90:2551-2555.
16. Gridley T, Soriano P, Jaenisch R et al. Insertional mutagenesis in mice. Trends in Genetics 1989; 3:162-166.

CHAPTER 9

New Perspectives for Antibody Therapeutics

INTRODUCTION

An ideal therapeutic antibody should have the following properties:

1) A specificity and affinity for the target sufficient to effect inactivation and/or removal of the target.

2) An in vivo biodistribution and serum half-life appropriate for the therapeutic regime.

3) A lack of cross reactivity with normal human tissues and components.

4) It should be immunosilent and suitable for repeated dosing and chronic application.

ANTIBODY AFFINITY AND SPECIFICITY

Humanized antibodies represent considerable progress towards the ideal antibody based therapeutic with a very low potential for immunogenicity, optimized human effector functions and an extended serum half-life. Specificity and affinity should also, in many cases, be optimal since the progenitor rodent monoclonal antibodies are normally selected as prime candidates from very extensive panels derived from immunized animals over many years of research.

This may not be the case, however, for a number of the anticancer monoclonal antibodies currently under clinical or preclinical evaluation. It is only in the past few years that a better understanding has been gained with respect to the properties required from an anti-tumor antibody. In order to achieve complement activation, radiation or toxin-driven removal of tumor cells it is desirable for the tumor surface to have a large number of antigen binding sites and it is preferable if the antigen has a functional role in the growth of cells. Epidermal growth factor receptors, for example, may have an antigen density as high as $3x10^6$ molecules per cell on carcinomas. Also, the target antigen should not be shed into the circulation in significant amounts. Many antibodies are rapidly internalized on binding to tumor surface antigen. This property is undesirable if it is hoped to activate human effector functions but desirable for delivery of toxins or drugs. Recent research has produced a new generation of anti-tumor antibodies which fulfill these criteria.[1-3]

The tacit assumption is often made that one should seek the highest affinity possible in the selection of a therapeutic antibody. However, this may not be the case. Effector function binding affinities for bivalent complement and FcR binding are of the order of $5x10^7$ M^{-1} and $5x10^8$ M^{-1} and hence there may be a saturation affinity for antigen-antibody interaction in vivo.

Circumstantial evidence suggests that a slow dissociation rate of antibody from antigen is more relevant for biological activity than affinity. Furthermore, where the target antigen is present in low abundance on normal body constituents, a high affinity antibody may increase potential for toxic side effects from antibody therapy. CAMPATH-1, one of the most effective antibody therapeutics, has a low affinity for its target antigen.

Biodistribution and Pharmacokinetics

Therapeutic IgG antibodies have extended serum half-lives of 14-21 days and about 45% of a therapeutic dose will diffuse into extravascular tissues. They are, therefore, ideal therapeutics for prophylaxis and treatment of infectious diseases, clearance of lymphoid tumor cells and many autoimmune disorders. However, they are not the optimal formulations for other clinical situations. In vivo imaging of organs or tumors requires more rapid blood and tissue clearance to reduce nonspecific binding and background interference. Also, penetration of solid tumors and deep-seated infections or passage across the blood–brain barrier will require different formulations.

Proteolytic digestion of intact immunoglobulin can only effectively generate Fab and $(Fab')_2$ fragments and these are currently used in formulations of in vivo imaging agents.

Genetic engineering technologies have now provided very extensive scope for antibody fragment formulations (Fig. 9.1) which can be manufactured directly in microbial cells.[4-6] A large body of data has already accumulated with respect to the properties of these fragment formulations and their pharmacokinetics in animals and man are being evaluated.[7-9] There is no doubt that many future therapeutics will be based upon antibody fragments manufactured in bacteria. Indeed, the first in vivo imaging studies have been described with bacterially produced single chain Fv against CEA.[10]

BIVALENT AND BIFUNCTIONAL ANTIBODY FRAGMENTS

Single chain Fvs (ScFv) are monomeric and often have reduced affinity for antigen due to lack of opportunity for avidity on binding. However, ScFv formulations often spontaneously assemble into dimeric $ScFv_2$ in bacteria.[11] These fragments act as simple chelating agents to block antigen function. They cannot recruit chemical signals or accessory cells to assist in destroying and removing the target.

A variety of bifunctional antibodies to target cellular cytotoxicity could be designed (Table 9.1) and a number of studies in animals have shown that targeting of cytotoxicity to tumors can be achieved.[12-14] Studies of bifunctional antibodies in humans have also demonstrated their efficacy[15,16] (chapter 4). Bifunctional antibodies to date have been made either chemically by coupling two Fab or from hybrid hybridomas, but these methods are not feasible for commercial production. However, methods for the direct assembly of bifunctional antibodies in both mammalian cells[17] and bacteria[18,19] have been described recently and one can expect an increasing effort devoted to bringing bifunctional antibodies forward to the clinic.

INTRACELLULAR ANTIBODIES

Monoclonal antibodies which internalize are taken up through clathrin coated pits by endocytosis and become trapped in the resulting internalized vesicles. Antibody-toxin/drug fusion products are so designed that the drug/toxin moiety is released from antibody by low pH or by proteolytic enzymes in such vesicles but

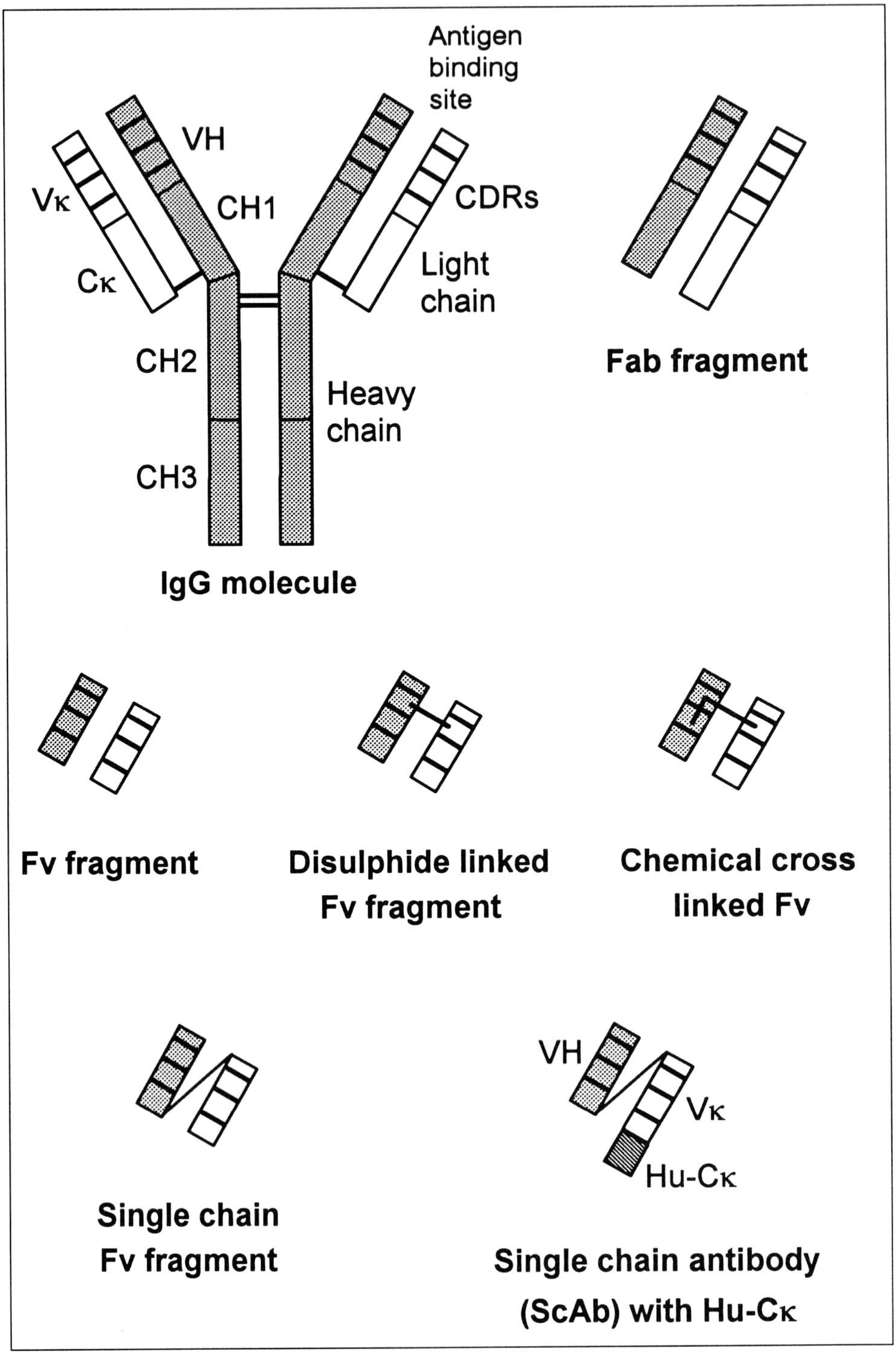

Fig. 9.1. IgG and its related antibody fragments. Many of these fragments have been successfully expressed as recombinant molecules from E. coli.

the antibody itself is not released into the cytoplasm of the cell. Intracellular targets cannot, therefore, be accessed by antibodies. However, a number of alternate methods of delivery are being investigated.

Our knowledge of peptide motifs within proteins which signal transport to particular intracellular compartments is increasing rapidly and it should be possible to attach appropriate motifs to antibodies to signal their release from endosomes into the cytoplasm.

The use of liposomes to deliver chemical drugs or vaccine antigens into the cytoplasm of cells is well established.[20] Antibody coated liposomes preferentially bind to the surface of cells containing the target antigen. Most types of liposomes enter the cell by endocytosis and the resulting endosome fuses with a lysosome to produce a phagolysosome wherein the lysososomal phospholipases degrade the liposome and release its contents. Antibody fragments would still remain trapped within such an organelle. However, pH-sensitive liposomes appear to fuse with the endosomal membrane and deliver their contents directly into the cytoplasm. This then may be a promising route to intracellular delivery of antibody fragments.

Genes encoding antibodies can be transfected into mammalian cells in vitro by standard methods of gene transfer.[21] In one example, genes encoding ScFv of anti-HIV-1 gp120 were introduced in vitro into HIV-infected T-lymphocytes and inhibited cell-cell fusion and HIV-1 production.[22] In vivo application, however, requires much more effective and specific methods of delivery and

Table 9.1. Formulations of bispecific antibodies which target cytotoxicity

Therapeutic target	Triggering molecule	Cytotoxic cells
Cancer	CD3	T cells
	CD44	T/NK cells
	TCR	T cells
	Ly-6C	T cells
	CD64(FcγR1)	PMN/monocytes
	CD69	NK cells
	CD16(FcγR111)	NK/macrophages
Infectious disease	FcγR11/R111	Macrophages/NK

one approach has been the incorporation of ScFv in retroviral vectors.[23] This offers the intriguing prospect of specificity of cell targeting through one antibody fragment displayed on the surface of the retrovirus and killing by intracellular delivery of a gene encoding a second antibody fragment.

Gene delivery should also prove of great value in the provision of transgenic 'knock-out' mice for drug research. A transgenic mouse carrying an antibody to inhibit expression of any target protein can be produced without any knowledge of the genetic locus of the target.

EXTENDING THE SCOPE AND IMMUNOSILENCE OF THERAPEUTIC ANTIBODIES

New technologies for generating human antibodies are reviewed in detail in earlier chapters. Figure 9.2 summarizes these methods and pinpoints the steps which may place limitations on the breadth of targets or level of immunosilence achievable.

It has proved very difficult to raise monoclonal antibodies against a number of desirable therapeutic targets through immunization (either in vivo or in vitro), in particular against self antigens, antigens with high amino acid sequence conservation across species and antigens which are involved in the development of the immune response itself. Phage technology offers a clear value in these cases.

All technologies carry potential for the persistence of, or introduction of, immunogenic epitopes. The first generation of humanized antibodies are well advanced in product development and are likely to be highly satisfactory therapeutics in a wide range of clinical situations. The residual potential for immunogencity may, however, limit their chronic use. In vitro mutagenesis is likely to be required during development of high affinity antibodies from both human phage libraries and SCID mouse technology with potential for the introduction of immunogenic domains. Synthetic and semisynthetic antibody phage libraries are abiotic and likely to prepossess immunogenic epitopes and it is unlikely that transgenic mice will screen out epitopes which will be immunogenic in man.

PEPTIDE MIMETICS OF ANTIBODIES

Although there is one report of a single VH polypeptide chain shown to retain significant antigen binding affinity[24] this has not proved to be a general phenomena. However, camel antibodies

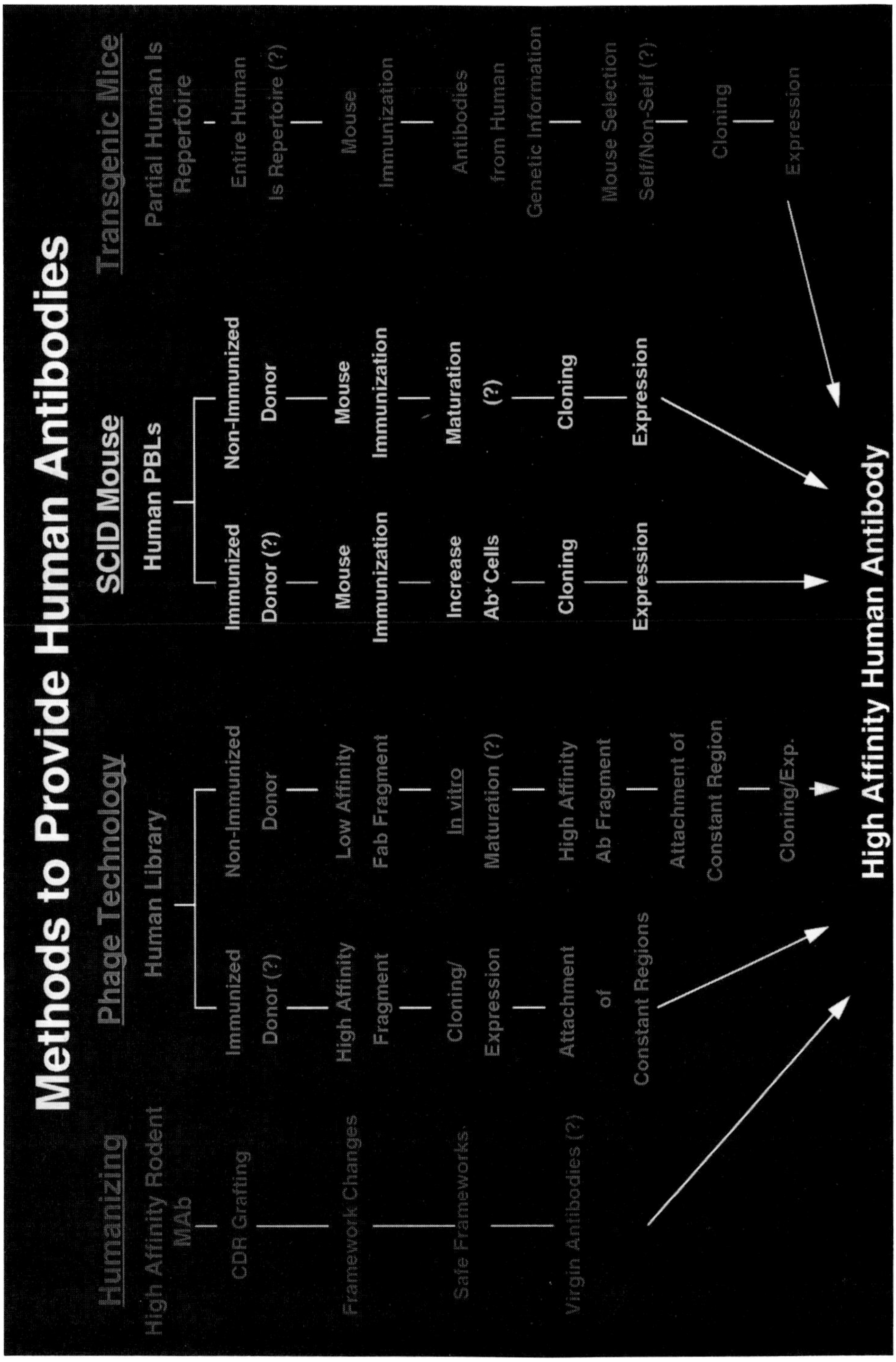

Fig. 9.2. New technologies for the provision of human antibodies.

occur naturally as VH structures only and they can have high binding affinity.[25] At present however, ScFv is the smallest fragment that reproducibly retains binding affinity equivalent to an intact antibody. There have been reports that single CDRs can independently retain sufficient binding affinity for practical application, and strategies using structural information of antigen antibody interactions to design peptide mimetics have been developed.[26]

SUMMARY

A new and exciting era in antibody based therapy is beginning and it is already clear that many products will be efficacious. Undoubtedly, limitations to the scope of these products will emerge but the plethora of new techniques will further extend their clinical use. There is enormous clinical and commercial value to be gained from the fact that these products, while treating a diverse range of infectious disease, cancer and autoimmunity, are essentially identical in all chemical, pharmacological and biological properties except those arising specifically from interaction with the target antigen. As a class, therefore, they are safe, non-toxic drugs whose in vivo properties are predictable from an early stage in research and development.

REFERENCES

1. Riethmuller G, Johnson JP. Monoclonal antibodies in the detection and therapy of micrometastatic epithelial cancers. Current Biology 1992; 4:647-655.
2. Rettig WJ, Garin-Chesa P, Healey JH et al. Identification of endosialin, a cell surface glycoprotein of vascular endothelial cells in human cancer. Proc Nat Acad Sci 1992; 89:10832-10836.
3. Kitamura K, Stockert E, Garin-Chesa P et al. Specificity analysis of blood group Lewis-y (Ley) antibodies generated against synthetic and natural Ley determinants. Proc Nat Acad Sci 1994; 91: 12957-12961.
4. Huston JS, McCartney J, Tai M-S et al. Medical applications of single chain antibodies. Int Rev Imunol 1993; 10:195-217.
5. Johnson S, Bird RE. Construction of single chain Fv derivatives of monoclonal antibodies and their production in *Escherichia coli*. Method Enzymol 1991; 203:88-98.
6. Pluckthun A. Antibodies from *Escherichia coli*. In: Rosenberg M, Moore GP eds. Therapeutic Pharmacology of Monoclonal Antibodies. Handbook of Pharmacology, Berlin: Springer Verlag 1994; 133:269-315.

7. Yokota T, Milenic DE, Whitlow M et al. Rapid tumour penetration of a single chain Fv and comparison with other immunoglobulin forms. Cancer Res 1992; 52:3402-3408.
8. Adams GP, McCartney JE, Tai M-S et al. Highly specific *in vivo* tumour targeting by monovalent and divalent forms of 741F8 anti-c-erb-2 single chain Fv. Cancer Res 1993; 53:4026-4034.
9. King DJ, Turner A, Farnsworth APH et al. Improved tumour targeting with chemically cross linked recombinant antibody fragments. Cancer Res 1994; 54:6176-6185.
10. Chester KA, Begent RH, Robson L et. al. Phage libraries for the generation of clinically useful antibodies. The Lancet. 1994; 343:455-457.
11. McGregor DP, Molloy PE, Cunningham C et al. Spontaneous assembly of bivalent single chain antibody fragments in *Escherichia coli.* Mol Immunol 1994; 31:219-226.
12. Barr IG, Miescher S, von Fliedner V et al. *In vivo* localisation of a bispecific antibody which targets human T lymphocytes to lyse human colon cancer cells. Int J Cancer 1989; 43:501-507.
13. Garrido MA, Valdayo MJ, Winkler DF et al. Targeting human T-lymphocytes with bispecific antibodies to react against human ovarian carcinoma cells growing in *nu/nu* mice. Cancer Res 1990; 50:4227-4232.
14. van Dijk J, Zegveld ST, Fleuren GJ et al. Localisation of monoclonal antibody G250 and bispecific monoclonal antibody CD3/G250 in human renal carcinoma xenografts: relative effects of size and affinity. Int J Cancer 1991; 48:738-743.
15. Mezzanzanica D, Canevari S, Colnaghi MI. Retargeting of human lymphocytes against human ovarian carcinoma cells by bispecific antibodies: from laboratory to clinic. Int J Clin Lab Res 199; 21:159-164.
16. Nitta T, Sato K, Yagita H et al. Preliminary trial of specific targeting therapy against malignant glioma. Lancet 1990; 335:368-371.
17. Hayden MS, Linsley PS, Gayle MA et al. Single-chain mono- and bispecific antibody derivatives with novel biological properties and antitumour activity from a COS cell transient expression system. Therap Immunol 1994; 1:3-15.
18. Carter P, Kelley RF, Rodrigues ML et al. High level *Escherichia coli* expression and production of a bivalent humanized antibody fragment. Biotechnology 1992; 10:163-167.
19. Hollliger P, Prospero T, Winter G. 'Diabodies': small bivalent and bispecific antibody fragments. Proc Nat Acad Sci 1993; 90: 6444-6448.
20. Gregoriadis G. Immunological adjuvants: a role for liposomes. Immunology Today 1990; 1:89-97.
21. Morgan DO, Roth RA. Analysis of intracellular protein function by antibody injection. Immunology Today 1988; 9:84-88.

22. Chen S-Y, Bagley J, Marasco WA. Intracellular antibodies as a new class of therapeutic molecules for gene therapy. Human Gene Therapy 1994; 5:595-601.
23. Russell SJ, Hawkins RE, Winter G. Retroviral vectors displaying functional antibody fragments. Nucleic Acid Res 1993; 21: 1081-1085.
24. Ward ES, Gussow D, Griffiths AD et al. Binding activities of a repertoire of single immunoglobulin variable domains secreted from *Escherichia coli.* Nature 1989; 341:544-546.
25. Muyldermans S, Atarbouch T, Saldanha J et al. Sequences and structure of VH domains from naturally occurring camel heavy chains in immunoglobulins lacking light chains. Protein Eng 1994; 7:1129-1135.
26. Dougall WC, Peterson NC, Greene MI. Antibody structure-based-design of pharmacological agents. Trends Biotech 1994: 12:372-378.

INDEX

Page numbers in italics denote figures (f) or tables (t).

Medical Intelligence Unit

Available and Upcoming Titles

- ❒ Hyperacute Xenograft Rejection
  Jeffrey Platt, Duke University
- ❒ Chimerism and Tolerance
  Suzanne Ildstad, University of Pittsburgh
- ❒ Birth Control Vaccines
  G.P. Talwar and Raj Raghupathy, National Institute of Immunology-New Delhi and University of Kuwait
- ❒ Monoclonal Antibodies in Transplantation
  Lucienne Chatenoud, Hôpital Necker-Paris
- ❒ Therapeutic Applications of Oligonucleotides
  Stanley Crooke, ISIS Pharmaceuticals
- ❒ Cryopreserved Venous Allografts
  Kelvin G.M. Brockbank, CryoLife, Inc.
- ❒ Clinical Benefits of Leukpodepleted Blood Products
  Joseph Sweeney and Andrew Heaton, Miriam and Roger Williams Hospitals-Providence and Irwin Memorial Blood Center-San Francisco
- ❒ Delta Hepatitis Virus
  M. Dinter-Gottlieb, Drexel University
- ❒ Intima Formation in Blood Vessels: Spontaneous and Induced
  Mark M. Kockx, Algemeen Ziekenhuis Middelheim-Antwerpen
- ❒ Adult T Cell Leukemia and Related Diseases
  Takashi Uchiyama and Jungi Yodoi, University of Kyoto
- ❒ Development of Epstein-Barr Virus Vaccines
  Andrew Morgan, University of Bristol
- ❒ p53 Suppressor Gene
  Tapas Mukhopadhyay, Steven Maxwell and Jack A. Roth, University of Texas-MD Anderson Cancer Center
- ❒ Sudden Death in Ischemic Heart Disease
  Malcolm D. Silver and Giorgio Baroldi, University of Toronto and University of Milan
- ❒ Minor Histocompatibility Antigens and Transplantation
  Craig V. Smith, University of Pittsburgh
- ❒ Familial Adenomatous Polyposis Coli and the APC Gene
  Joanna Groden, University of Cincinnati
- ❒ Cancer Cell Adhesion and Tumor Invasion
  Pnina Brodt, McGill University
- ❒ Constitutional Immunity to Infection
  Cees M. Verduin, David A. Watson, Jan Verhoef, Hans Van Dijk, University of Utrecht and North Dakota State University
- ❒ Nutritional and Metabolic Support in Critically Ill Patients
  Rifat Latifi and Stanley Dudrick, Yale University
- ❒ Nutritional Support in Gastrointestinal Failure
  Rifat Latifi and Stanley Dudrick, Yale University
- ❒ Septic Myocardiopathy: Molecular Mechanisms
  Karl Werdan, Ludwig-Maximilians-Universität-München
- ❒ The Molecular Genetics of Wilms Tumor
  Max Coppes, Christine Campbell and Bryan R.G. Williams, Cleveland Clinic and University of Calgary
- ❒ Endothelins
  David J. Webb and Gillian Gray, University of Edinburgh
- ❒ Nutritional and Metabolic Support in Cancer, Transplant and Immunocompromised Patients
  Rifat Latifi, Yale University
- ❒ Antibody-Mediated Graft Rejection
  J. Andrew Bradley and Eleanor Bolton, University of Glasgow
- ❒ Liposomes in Cancer Chemotherapy
  Steven Sugarman, University of Texas-MD Anderson
- ❒ Molecular Basis of Human Hypertension
  Florent Soubrier, Collége de France-Paris
- ❒ Endocardial Endothelium: Control of Cardiac Performance
  Stanislas U. Sys and Dirk Brutsaert, Universiteit Antwerpen
- ❒ Endovascular Stented Grafts for the Treatment of Vascular Diseases
  Michael L. Marin, Frank J. Veith and Barry A. Levine, Albert Einstein College of Medicine
- ❒ B Cells and Autoimmunity
  Christian Boitard, Hôpital Necker-Paris
- ❒ Immunity to Mycobacteria
  Ian Orme, Colorado State University
- ❒ Hepatic Stem Cells and the Origin of Hepatic Carcinoma
  Stewart Sell, University of Texas-Houston
- ❒ HLA and Maternal-Fetal Recognition
  Joan S. Hunt, University of Kansas
- ❒ Transplantation Tolerance
  J. Wesley Alexander, University of Cincinnati
- ❒ Ovarian Autoimmunity
  Roy Moncayo and Helga E. Moncayo, University of Innsbruck
- ❒ Ex Vivo Cell Therapy for Cancer
  Ronald Herberman, University of Pittsburgh
- ❒ Protein and Amino Acid Metabolism in Cancer
  Peter W.T. Pisters and Murray Brennan, Sloan-Kettering Memorial Cancer Center
- ❒ Cytokines and Hemorrhagic Shock
  Eric J. DeMaria, Medical College of Virginia
- ❒ Endometriosis
  Lisa Barrie Schwartz, New York University and David Olive, Yale University
- ❒ T Cell Vaccination and Autoimmune Disease
  Jingwu Zhang, Willems Institut-Belgium
- ❒ Immune Privilege
  J. Wayne Streilein, Luke Jiang and Bruce Ksander, Schepens Eye Research Institute-Boston
- ❒ The Pathophysiology of Sepsis and Multi-Organ Failure
  Mitchell Fink, Harvard University
- ❒ Bone Metastasis
  F. William Orr, McMaster University
- ❒ Novel Regional Therapies for Liver Tumors
  Seiji Kawasaki and Masatoshi Makuuchi, Shinshu University
- ❒ Thyroid Hormone Resistance
  Roy E. Weiss and Michael Refetoff, University of Chicago
- ❒ Growth Hormone in Critical Illness
  Michael Torosian, University of Pennsylvania
- ❒ Molecular Biology of Aneurysms
  Richard R. Keen, Northwestern University
- ❒ Strategies in Malaria Vaccine Design
  F.E.G. Cox, King's College London
- ❒ Chimeric Proteins and Fibrinolysis
  Christoph Bode, Marschall Runge and Edgar Haber, University of Heidelberg, University of Texas-Galveston and Harvard University

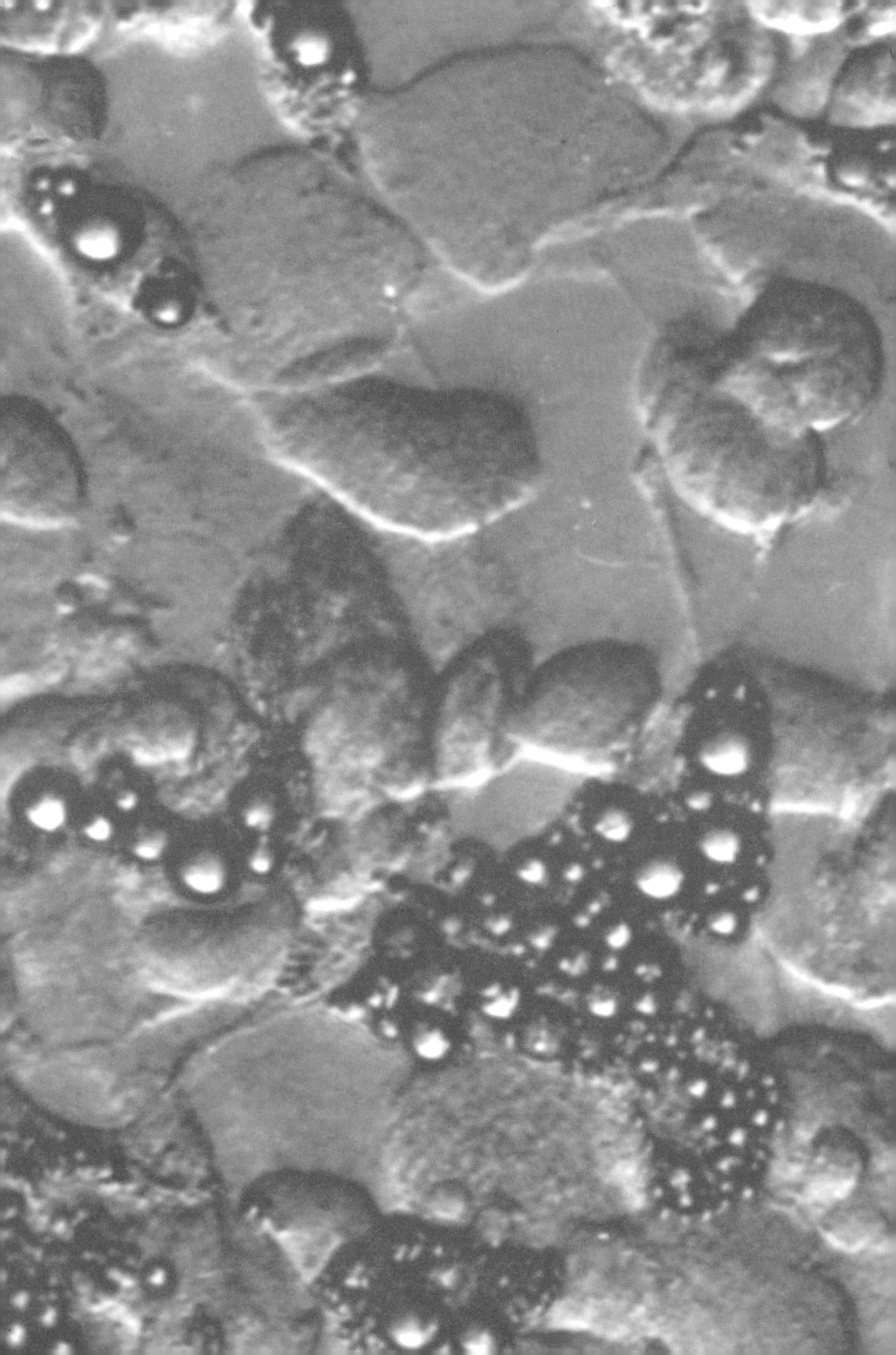